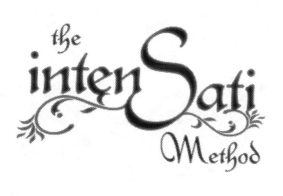

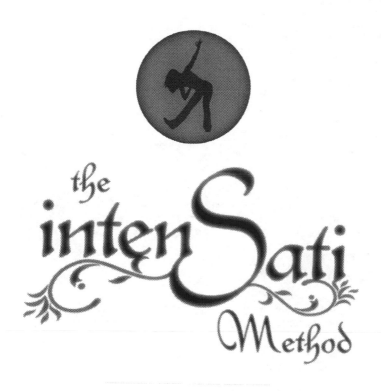

THE SEVEN SECRET PRINCIPLES TO THINNER PEACE

PATRICIA MORENO

Simon Spotlight Entertainment

NEW YORK LONDON TORONTO SYDNEY

NOTE TO READERS
This publication contains the opinions and ideas of its author. It is intended to provide helpful and informative material on the subjects addressed in the publication. It is sold with the understanding that the author and publisher are not engaged in rendering medical, health, or any other kind of personal professional services in the book. The reader should consult his or her medical, health, or other competent professional before engaging in any exercise program or adopting any of the suggestions in this book or drawing inferences from it.

The author and publisher specifically disclaim all responsibility for any liability, loss, or risk, personal or otherwise, which is incurred as a consequence, directly or indirectly, of the use and application of any of the contents of this book.

 Simon Spotlight Entertainment
A Division of Simon & Schuster, Inc.
1230 Avenue of the Americas
New York, NY 10020

First Simon Spotlight Entertainment hardcover edition January 2010

SIMON SPOTLIGHT ENTERTAINMENT and colophon are trademarks of Simon & Schuster, Inc.

For information about special discounts for bulk purchases, please contact Simon & Schuster Special Sales at 1-866-506-1949 or business@simonandschuster.com.

The Simon & Schuster Speakers Bureau can bring authors to your live event. For more information or to book an event, contact the Simon & Schuster Speakers Bureau at 1-866-248-3049 or visit our website at www.simonspeakers.com.

Designed by Jaime Putorti

Manufactured in the United States of America

10 9 8 7 6 5 4 3 2 1

Library of Congress Cataloging-in-Publication Data
Moreno, Patricia.
The IntenSati method : the seven secret principles to thinner peace / Patricia Moreno.
p. cm.
1. Weight loss. 2. Health. 3. Mind and body. I. Title.
RM222.2.M5685 2009
613.2'5–dc22   2009021807

ISBN 978-1-4391-5298-0

To all those who have stopped
believing in themselves . . .
and are ready to change their mind.

CONTENTS

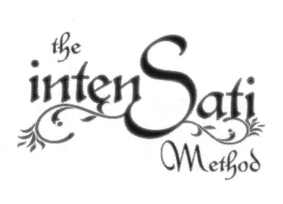

INTRODUCTION

I have struggled for most of my life with weight, eating disorders, diets, and different workouts, always looking for the answer to my problem. Yet I could never find the magic pill, the perfect diet, the exercise of all exercises. What I have found is that most anything will work . . . if you can get yourself to do it. It is not the diet that fails, but the willpower that fails. It is not that an exercise doesn't work for your body type; it is that you can't get yourself to commit to doing it consistently, or you're simply not motivated enough to start.

I come from a family of eleven kids: eight girls and three boys. In my home, there were always huge amounts of food—and no discipline or rules. So I ate whatever I wanted, as much as I wanted, whenever I wanted—wonderful Mexican food and all the popular American junk foods: doughnuts, sodas, cookies, ice cream. By the time I was fifteen, I weighed 212 pounds! Then came diets, diet pills, fasts, liquid diets; you name it, I did it all. Whenever I was on a diet I would lose weight, and whenever I wasn't I would gain it all back . . . and then some. I started teaching aerobics in high school and got down to 140 pounds, but over the years my weight always fluctuated by 30 or so pounds.

I also battled bulimia, the dreadful binge-and-purge cycle, and exercise addiction. It moved me into a depression and a deeper self-loathing; I was a fitness professional who was not living a very healthy life, and I had a secret that I didn't want anyone to find out. My guilt around food got so bad that even eating a bowl of lettuce would send a tidal wave of shame over me.

The secret grew, the guilt and shame grew, and my perspective of myself worsened every day. I had managed to increase my workouts to five to eight solid hours a day. It was the only way I could manage myself. One day I finally opened up to a good friend, sharing all my struggles around food, exercise, and body image. As soon as I told her about my secret pain, the healing began. I found a therapist who specialized in eating disorders, Dr. Judith Brissman, and over the course of a few years she helped me recover from bulimia. With her guidance, I found my way out of the darkest and loneliest period of my life. And here is where my longing for a better way began.

The journey has been a long and challenging one. I have spent every single day of my life since the third grade looking for solutions to my love-hate relationship with food and my body. This book has come about after more than twenty years in the fitness industry and my personal quest for freedom around issues of my body, my weight, my self-esteem, and my happiness. I have read much, studied voraciously, prayed, meditated, and searched for answers to the question "How do I get myself to where I want to be, both thin *and* happy?" I had been thin before, but the joy was still painfully missing from my life. I had successful workout programs, popular classes, a TV show. I was sponsored by clothing and shoe companies; I was in magazines, aerobics competitions, and ad campaigns. I trained thousands of instructors all over the world. I studied dance, yoga, martial arts, meditation, life coaching, and nutrition, but I still couldn't find the key to happiness. So I sought to figure it out myself. And I did.

Before your journey begins, there is some work to do. Maybe you have tried a million other diets before and failed. I hear you. This one is different, and you will have to do something differently if you want a different result. Do you know one definition of *insanity*? Doing the same thing over and over and expecting a new outcome. My program is the answer to that insanity. It is a unique, holistic approach to dieting and fitness. I will guide you through mental, physical, and spiritual exercises that will help you become who you really want to be. This is a spiritual approach to weight loss, and you will not only lose the pounds but gain clarity and purpose. You will gain both inner and thinner peace!

This program, called IntenSati, teaches you how to use your conscious, goal-making mind to access and awaken your spiritual or subconscious mind, the part of your mind that holds your beliefs about yourself, your personality, and the driving center of your actions. Ultimately we can set all the goals we want, but until we take action, we are just big talkers and will continue fueling the belief that it is too hard or impossible to have the life and body we want. You have everything you need right now within you to fulfill any goal; this program helps you awaken and channel that power.

My belief in the power of the mind was instilled in me at a very early age. My father was a firm believer in it. He read endless books on the subject; I remember him always having one book in his pocket and one in his hand. I believe that his interest in the power of the mind may have not only saved my life but instilled in me an understanding of the power of our thoughts at a very early age.

At twelve, I was diagnosed with a bone marrow infection in my right arm. I was in the hospital for about two weeks and the drugs I was being given were not making a difference. The doctors told my parents they were worried the infection would spread to my heart and be fatal. They planned to do an exploratory surgery and they told my parents that there was a possibility they would have to amputate my arm. I didn't know about any of these conversations until afterward.

The night before the surgery my father came to my room after everyone had left. He sat by my bed and he told me a story. He had me close my eyes and imagine an army of soldiers, each dressed in their uniforms and carrying various tools, like shovels and picks. He had me envision this little army marching into my arm and finding the infection and shoveling it out. After they shoveled the infection out, they hosed the arm clean, then put everything back together and marched out. He mentally led me moment by moment through the whole process. I am not sure how long he sat by my side and we engaged in this visualization, but by the morning the infection was gone. The surgery was canceled, and soon I was released from the hospital.

For years I forgot about the incident, but when I began developing the intenSati method, this memory came flooding back to me, as vivid as if it had happened yesterday. What it shows me is that the power of the mind can do anything; it can, as it did for me, turn your health around and save your life. I know it is not easy to change the way you think. It takes discipline and practice as well as a deep level of self-love and self-respect because you have to *own* your power.

This book is about taking care of you, all parts of you: your mind, your spirit, and your body. This practice is a way of life. This is an awakening, a new beginning, an act of love and kindness, willpower, courage, compassion, and grace. There is no body that cannot get healthier. There is no mind that cannot become clearer. And there is no spirit that cannot overcome the greatest of challenges to find love and joy. So come with me and get ready to transform yourself into the person you know you can become.

WHAT IS THE
INTENSATI METHOD?

always felt there was a missing link in the fitness programs out there: the link between mind and body. No matter what type of exercise you do, part of the process is nonphysical. I believe that to transform yourself, you have to train not only your body but also your mind, your concentration, and your focus. Inten derives from "intention," and Sati is a Pali word that means "mindfulness." IntenSati is like no workout you have ever experienced. It fuses high-energy aerobics, martial arts, dance, yoga, and strength conditioning with meditation, positive psychology, and quantum physics. And while it sounds complex, it is so very simple: IntenSati combines spoken affirmations with simple choreography to build physical, mental, and spiritual muscle.

I felt a strong desire within me to create something that would really make a difference in people's lives, something that would motivate those who were having trouble achieving their goals. Most of my students in New York City were young, successful, type-A people who loved a challenge and did not need to be motivated to get to the gym. But I knew this wasn't the norm;

I wanted to create a practice for someone who doesn't like exercise or has trouble sticking to a regular workout regime. On a personal level, I wanted to create something for my family, my sisters and brothers who were having trouble losing weight and keeping it off. This would be a workout that could work for anyone, at any age, and at any level of fitness; it would help people change how they think, move, speak, and act on a daily basis.

I call IntenSati a *practice* because it is an opportunity for anyone to practice feeling good, empowered, courageous, enthusiastic, passionate, focused, confident, happy, and in love. These are powerful positive emotions. After you practice feeling good and you know you can choose it, you will never be the same again.

In a traditional workout class, your body is going through the motions but your mind is on other things. You could be thinking about how much longer you have to endure this workout. Maybe you're thinking, "I'm dying . . . only five more minutes and I'm outta here!" or "I have so much I need to get done at work this afternoon." There is no way you can do your best while your mind is somewhere else and full of complaints. Even worse, you are not likely to continue with something you don't enjoy. IntenSati is the first workout that fuses the power of positive thinking with physical exercise.

A New Name for Exercise

In IntenSati, you won't find exercises called lunge, crunch, or squat. Instead, you'll be doing exercises called Courage, Strength, and Faith, for example. The exercises are named for the attitude you are embodying, because the goal is to focus on training your emotions. In the following chapters, you will learn how to embody the statements with movements that will start to change you on a cellular level. Thoughts fuel your emotions, and motion fuels your emotions. So when you combine thought with action, your emotions will give you strength, courage, and stamina—all you need to make the right choices and hold tight to your vision.

Each exercise is broken down into three parts: the Action, the Attitude, the Affirmation. The Action is what you are doing with your body (the way you move your arms or legs or stand). The Attitude is the expression of your heart—the emotion. The Affirmation is the mental exercise, or what you are saying. For example, when you do the exercise Strength, the action is a punch, the attitude is strength, and the affirmation is "I am strong."

The IntenSati Vocabulary

Before you begin the IntenSati practice, it will be helpful for you to understand the power of each pose and its meaning, both in word and in action. You will see these poses frequently in the IntenSati exercises that appear in the book. Review this section carefully; practice each word by saying it, doing it (through the pose), and embodying it. Eventually, you will memorize these poses, but refer back to these pages if you need a refresher.

1. BEAUTY

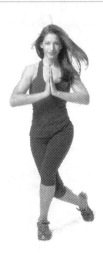

ACTION: Step your right foot slightly behind and back across your left foot. Keeping the left foot planted on the floor, allow the right heel to rise as you bend your knees to a cross lunge. Square your hips front and center, keeping the back straight and abs in. Your palms are pressing together in front of the heart in the Prayer position.

AFFIRMATION: "I am beautiful."

ATTITUDE: This pose allows you to practice looking for the good and the beauty in yourself, your life, and others. The bowing forward action inspires a softening of the heart, humility, and gentleness. Feel your heart open as you experience more joy, more love, more appreciation for the world around you.

2. COMPASSION

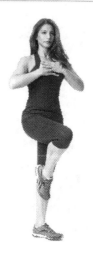

ACTION: Stand on your left leg, bend your right leg, and place your right foot by your left knee, in a single-leg balance. Place your palms across your heart.

AFFIRMATION: "I am compassionate."

ATTITUDE: Buddha said, "Compassion is that which makes the heart of the Good move at the pain of others." When we cultivate compassion for ourselves, we are cultivating self-love. When we have self-love, we are more capable of loving others. As you place your hands on your heart with this gesture, feel the love you are offering to yourself. Let your compassionate heart be your gift to yourself, others, and all of life.

3. COURAGE

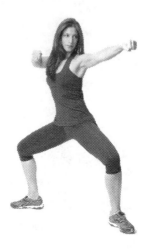

ACTION: Stand with feet together, placing the right forearm over the left forearm in front of your body. Step to the back, diagonal with the right foot, into a Warrior stance (feet turned out in a V-position and knees bent and tracking over the ankles). With your fists and palms facing down, simultaneously straighten your left arm directly to your side and slide your right fist by your shoulder as if you were shooting a bow and arrow. Your back is straight, your pelvis tucked under, and your abs in.

AFFIRMATION: "I am courageous."

ATTITUDE: It takes courage not to settle for mediocrity but to go for greatness. Every time you do this exercise, feel the opening of your heart and the directing of your intention (like an arrow flying at its target!) with passion. Yes, you will be faced with challenge, but just as any warrior knows her path will demand courage, know that yours will, too, and the reward will be a happier and healthier life.

4. DESIRE

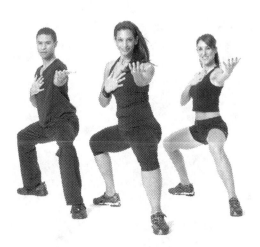

ACTION: Stand with your feet hip width apart and bend your knees. Make a triangle with your thumb and index fingers. Place your right hand on your heart and then extend both your arms out and in as quickly as possible. Hold your abs in and keep your back straight.

AFFIRMATION: "I want it! I want it! I really, really want it!"

ATTITUDE: I call desire the fire of transformation! When you really want something, that powerful energy within you propels you forward, gives you courage, and ignites the passion in your heart. If you really, really want to live a life you love in a body you love, you will find a way. Do you really, really want it?

5. FAITH

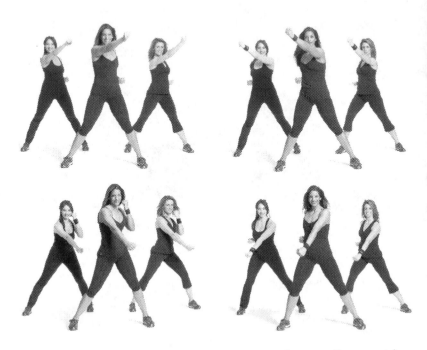

ACTION: Assume the Warrior stance. Bend your elbows with your fists at either side of your chin. Powerfully punch two times up and diagonally across your body, then two times down and diagonally across your body. It is up/up, down/down.

AFFIRMATION: "I believe I will succeed."

ATTITUDE: Faith is a choice, and it is a must if you are going to succeed. Faith is the cornerstone of a thriving life and body. Mother Teresa was quoted as saying, "I don't pray for success, I pray for faithfulness." All you need is a little faith, and that is the doorway to success.

6. FEARLESS

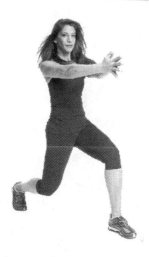

ACTION: Stand with your feet together and your palms pressing together and touching your heart, in the Prayer position. Take a large step forward with the left foot and bend your knees in a front lunge. Remember to keep your front foot flat on the floor and your knee tracking over your ankle and let the heel of your left foot come off the floor. Tuck your pelvis under while keeping your back straight and your abs in. Remain in the lunge position and extend your arms straight out in front of you, palms pressing together.

AFFIRMATION: "I am fearless now."

ATTITUDE: We cannot control all the circumstances of our life, but we can become stronger in facing the challenges that we encounter. Being fearless is about learning to face those challenges and fears instead of becoming paralyzed by them. When you take action in spite of your fear, you gain self-confidence and courage.

7. GRATITUDE

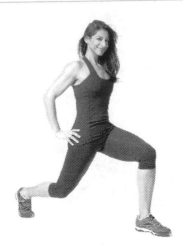

ACTION: Step your right foot behind you to a rear lunge, keeping your left foot flat on the floor and your right heel raised. Keep your back straight, your pelvis tucked under, and your abs in. Your hands are on your hips.

AFFIRMATION: "I am grateful now."

ATTITUDE: If there is one attitude that can change your life in an instant, gratitude is it. Think of how you feel when you are experiencing deep thankfulness for someone or something in your life. Feel the emotion that wells up inside of you if you let it. That emotion can shift your life, because you cannot feel hate, anger, envy, unworthiness, or depression when you feel gratitude. If you can practice feeling grateful, you will soon have more to be grateful for.

8. HAPPY

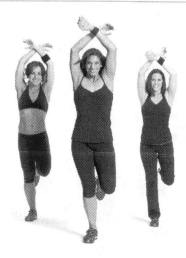

ACTION: Circle your arms away from you in giant sweeping arcs as you alternate feet, kicking yourself in the butt.

AFFIRMATION: "I am happier now."

ATTITUDE: Make happiness easy to achieve by making it unconditional. Make it your goal in spite of your circumstances. Happiness is a choice; practice choosing it every day. When you do this exercise, try to express outrageous, absurd happiness for absolutely no reason! Feel the joy circling you as you circle your arms in the air; the kick in the butt is the reminder to have fun and stop complaining!

9. INSPIRED

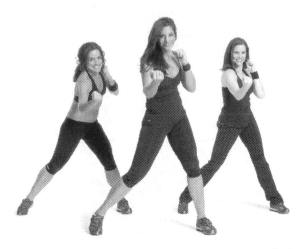

ACTION: In both martial arts and boxing, this is called an upper cut. Stand with your feet hip distance apart. Make a strong fist with both hands. Rotate and reach one fist up in front but away from your face while the opposite hand stays at chin level.

AFFIRMATION: "I am inspired now."

ATTITUDE: When you feel inspired, you are unstoppable. You will knock out any doubt, fear, or worry that is blocking you from taking action toward your goal. You cannot be doubtful and inspired at the same time. If you want to succeed, you need to practice finding ways to stay inspired! How does it feel to be inspired? How do you move when you are inspired? Feel it when you do this exercise. Act as if, and soon you will be.

10. INTENTION

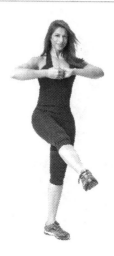

ACTION: Balance on your left leg, and raise your right foot to knee height. Bend your elbows and link your fingers in front of your heart. Pull your hands away from each other to activate your upper back muscles. With focused intention, straighten your right leg in front of you.

AFFIRMATION: "I claim my power to intend."

ATTITUDE: You can intend the direction you want your life to go in, but it is awe-inspiring when you deliberately do it and see the results. Your extended leg and foot represent the absolute clarity of your intention. You are pointing with purpose; you know exactly what you want. Your hands in gratitude symbolize your faith that your intention is already complete and on its way.

11. LOVE

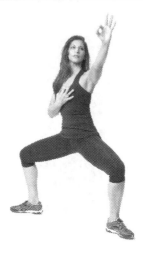

ACTION: Step diagonally to the back with your right foot into the Warrior stance. Create two circles by joining your thumb and index finger. Place your right palm over your heart, extend your left arm forward, and gaze through the circle like a keyhole.

AFFIRMATION: "I love myself."

ATTITUDE: Love refers to a variety of emotions, attitudes, and feelings. It is both a noun and a verb. It is very difficult to describe, but everyone knows what it feels like to be in love, to be loving, and to be loved, and we know the absence of it is painful. This pose reminds you that love is always present. The more you give love, the more you receive it, and if you are feeling a lack of it in your life, all you have to do is be loving. The hand gesture in this pose is the "OK" sign, and it symbolizes your willingness to see yourself and the world through the eyes of love. When you do, everything will be "OK."

12. PEACE

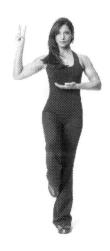

ACTION: Stand on your left foot and bring your right foot up to knee height to a single-leg balance. Extend your forearms parallel to the floor, bend your right elbow, and make a "peace" sign with your right hand. Cup your left hand just below your heart and stand tall.

AFFIRMATION: "I am peaceful now."

ATTITUDE: Surrender hostility toward yourself and others, and remember that peace is a choice. We can find it by letting go of worry, doubt, and fear. Worrying is like praying for what you don't want, and choosing peace will set you free. When you do this pose, breathe deeply and feel your commitment to inner peace rising.

13. POWER

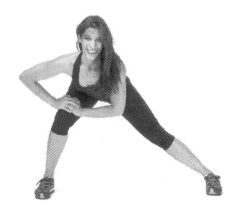

ACTION: Take a wide step to the left to a deep, powerful lunge, bending your right knee deeply and keeping your left knee straight. Your back is straight, and your feet are parallel. Place both hands on your right thigh for support.

AFFIRMATION: "I am powerful now."

ATTITUDE: Authentic power means leading your life knowing who you truly are in the highest sense. You are blessed with the power to think, to love, to will, to imagine, to plan, to create. You also have the power to hate, to doubt, to complain, to worry, to fear, and to discourage yourself. But the greatest power of all is your free will to choose. When you do this pose, let it always remind you of how powerful you are.

14. READY

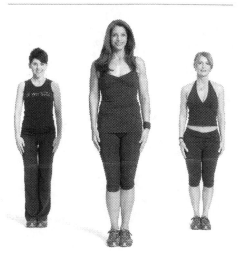

ACTION: Stand with your feet together, legs strong, chest lifted, and arms down by your sides.

AFFIRMATION: "I am ready now."

ATTITUDE: Declaring that you are ready to take on the challenge of changing your life, your mind, your body, or your emotional state is the first step toward success. A state of readiness implies that you are in the present moment and willing to do your best.

15. SELF-CONTROL

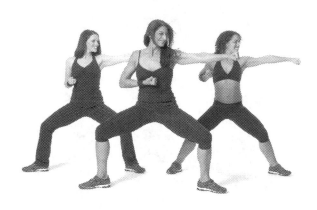

ACTION: Stand with your feet wider than hip width apart and bend your knees until your thighs are parallel to the floor. Cross your left arm over your right as if you are hugging yourself. Then extend your left arm to the side as if you are blocking something. In martial arts this is called a side block.

AFFIRMATION: "I have self-control."

ATTITUDE: Self-control is essential if you are on a journey of personal empowerment, weight loss, or transformation. It is the ability to say "No, I will not do that anymore" and be able to follow through. This takes practice and a strong will. It is a must if you want to change your life or your body.

16. STRENGTH

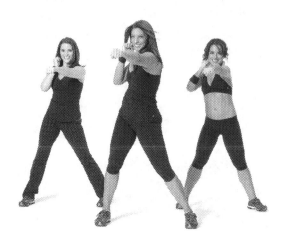

ACTION: Stand with your feet hip width apart, your elbows bent and close to your body, your fists at either side of your chin, in the On-Guard position. Punch your right fist across your body, palm facing down, allowing your torso to rotate slightly. Return to the On-Guard position. Repeat on the other side. Remember to keep your elbows pointing toward the floor and palms facing down. Return to the On-Guard position after each punch.

AFFIRMATION: "I am strong now."

ATTITUDE: Declare your strengths, and they will get stronger; don't focus on what you can't do. Remind yourself that you are strong enough to handle any challenge you are faced with right now. Use this exercise to remind you that you are strong enough, and embody that strength by doing your best!

17. SURRENDER

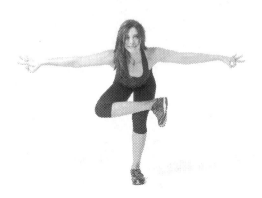

ACTION: Standing on your left leg, place your right ankle over your left knee. Take a deep single-leg squat, bending deeply from your knees and hips. Bend forward with your back straight. Extend your arms wide on either side of your body. Bring your thumbs and index fingers together to create circles.

AFFIRMATION: "I surrender now."

ATTITUDE: This pose reminds us of the power of letting go. When you take this pose, you are *allowing* life to be, instead of forcing it to be what you want it to be. This helps you move out of the mental state of fear, for when you embody "surrender," you are also embodying faith and trust in the universal laws and in your power to cocreate. This pose can bring great relief.

18. VICTORY

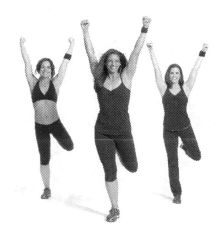

ACTION: Jog or march in place and enthusiastically reach your arms up in a wide V-position. Look upward and place the huge smile of a winner on your face, knowing that victory is yours.

AFFIRMATION: "I am victorious now."

ATTITUDE: If you can hold the attitude of a winner, think and move like a winner, success *must* be yours! When you do this exercise, feel the success, the joy, the achievement, and celebrate it before it shows up.

19. WARRIOR

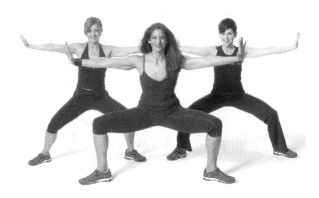

ACTION: Stand with your feet wider than hip width apart and bend your knees until your thighs are parallel to the floor. Make sure your feet are flat on the floor and your knees are over your ankles. Extend both arms powerfully out to the sides as if you are pushing two walls away from you.

AFFIRMATION: "I am a warrior now."

ATTITUDE: This is a very courageous pose. When we are afraid, we protect ourselves by closing down and covering ourselves up. The Warrior pose is the opposite. Doing this pose and embodying the spirit of a warrior will shift your emotional state from powerless to powerful.

20. YES

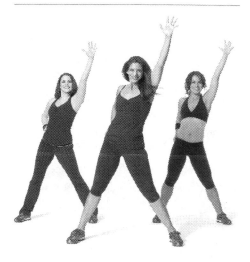

ACTION: Stand with your feet a little wider than hip width apart. Reach enthusiastically upward, alternating arms. Spread your fingers wide open so they look happy and alive!

AFFIRMATION: "Yes!" I am committed now."

ATTITUDE: When you say yes to your dream and you commit to fulfilling your goal no matter what, you will have access to all the things you need to fulfill your destiny. It begins with your level of commitment. How committed are you to feeling good now?

BASIC MEDITATION

Meditation is the practice of turning inward, a way of bringing yourself into the power of the present moment. There are many ways to meditate. I learned transcendental meditation many years ago, and it has truly been one of the most important practices of my life. In the practice of transcendental meditation, you repeat a phrase or a mantra in your mind. This allows your mind to become more quiet and still. Many people say they don't know how to meditate, yet every time you daydream, you are meditating. You can start a simple meditation practice for just a few minutes a day. Just be still and allow your mind to settle down. The best times to meditate are when you wake up in the morning and you are still a little sleepy or after a stretch, yoga, or IntenSati workout.

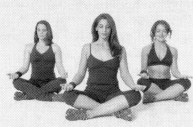 Sit in a comfortable position in a chair or on a pillow with your legs crossed and your palms resting on your thighs. Gently close your eyes and begin to slow down your breath. Hold a phrase mentally—"I Am" while you inhale and "Here" when you exhale. Do this for a few minutes until the affirmation just fades away and you feel yourself in a more peaceful state. Stay there as long as possible. After a few moments you may begin to hold in your mind the vision of your intention already fulfilled. See yourself happy, healthy, peaceful, and successful. Create a clear vision in your mind of yourself having already achieved your goal. Think *from* that place of success instead of thinking *about* it. When you take the time to do this, even if it is for just three to five minutes, you will notice a significant increase in your energy level, your peace of mind, and your ability to achieve difficult things. 🔲

PATRICIA MORENO

principle one

AS SOON AS YOU MAKE THE DECISION TO CHANGE, YOUR LIFE WILL FOLLOW

Think about it: if you want to go someplace new, if you want to change your horizons, you cannot get there by standing still. Maybe you feel that you're at a roadblock. You want to be someone else, someone happier, fitter, healthier, stronger. But just *wishing* for change is not enough; you have to take the first step. You have to find the power within you that will move you in the direction you want to go.

If you want your life to change from the course it is on, *you* must be willing to change. Not the circumstances, not someone else, not your parents or your spouse or your boss. It may be a word, an exercise, or an affirmation; all you need is a spark, something that will make you think differently than you have before. Somewhere in this book you will find something that will change your life.

Principle 1 of the IntenSati Method is that as soon as you make the decision to change, your life will follow. It has to. You are the one directing it. You are doing it every second of every minute of every hour of every day of every year till death do you part. *That* is power! To change physically, you have to be willing to change the way you think, feel, and act. The thoughts you are thinking, whether you are paying attention to them or not, are activating emotions within you. Those emotions fuel your energy, and that energy fuels your actions. IntenSati is the practice of keeping your attention on your thoughts, guiding them and your self-talk *deliberately* to activate emotions that will empower you instead of disempower you. It will enable you to live a life in which you are appreciating, loving, creating, and caring, instead of complaining and worrying most of the time.

Now, usually, when we know we need to change something, we think about the actions we're going to change. "I'm going to start going to the gym three times a week to get rid of this tummy!" we'll say, or "I'm going to start cooking healthier meals and reduce my calorie count," in the hope that these actions will turn us into thinner, happier people. It's a nice plan, but how many times have you started a new program only to find yourself in the same place a few weeks, a few months, or a few years later? It takes an extraordinary amount of mindfulness and desire to take inspired action. Your success starts well before the trip to the grocery store or your first jog around the block. Before you do anything, you have to pay attention to what is inspiring your actions (or your lack of them). You have to take control of your thoughts and mind and first understand the person you *really* are and the power you have to ignite powerful, positive, loving emotions.

Words to live by

Your positive loving thought is the highest form of prayer.

Keep your thoughts on the good you desire.

Worrying is like praying for what you don't want.

PATRICIA MORENO

You Are the Thinker, Not the Thought

If you have been hating yourself, loathing your body, or criticizing your lack of willpower and courage to change, it is precisely that inner conversation that is holding you back. It's robbing you of your power. Think of every thought you have not as an observation, but as a command. Most of us don't even notice or question the thoughts we have. But the fact is, you are what you think about all day long.

If you have the belief that you cannot lose weight, that no matter what you do you will fail, then guess what? You will fail. If you feel that weight on your body is stubborn and will never go away, then it will obey. Why? It is not the condition that is stubborn. *You* are stubbornly holding a thought that is keeping that condition in place. Think about how you speak about your body and what you tell your friends and family. Do you say things like:

* *"It's impossible for me to lose weight."*
* *"No matter what I do, I can't stick to a diet."*
* *"I hate exercise and I can't find something I like to do."*
* *"I am lazy. I have no willpower."*
* *"I give up! Diets don't work for me."*

Now look back at those words not as observations, but as commands. You are the one in charge. Why can't you lose weight, stick to a diet, or find a workout that works? Because *you* have been telling yourself—and probably anyone who will listen—how powerless, helpless, and hopeless you are. And so it is!

Let Your Heart Be Your Guide

You *can* change your life. No matter how far you think you've gone astray, you can get back on track starting *this moment*. First, you need to start paying attention to your thoughts. Will you make a commitment to yourself and catch yourself when you feel that negative feeling bubbling? Use those nagging, needling words that pop into your head and your heart as your red flag. Let them guide you to get back on track. When you hear them or feel them creeping up on you, stop, refocus, and choose to replace them with something more powerful and constructive. If you do this, you will begin to see yourself differently. Other people will see you differently. You will begin to wake up to a whole new world of possibilities.

Try this exercise. What if, instead of those negative things you tell yourself day after day, you try verbalizing the following thoughts instead? Say them out loud, whisper them, write them, feel them, imagine them as your truth. When one feels particularly good to you, use it. If it brings up a positive emotion, summon it like a prayer, repeating it over and over. Feel it create a change of focus within you. It's like turning on a light switch! When you turn on the light, all the dark disappears. This is the beginning of creating a new script for the New You. When you have a new script, you will have a new life.

As you read the lines below, take a few moments to imagine what powerful actions would follow these powerful statements of responsibility. This is the beginning . . .

* ❋ *"I can change now; I am ready."*
* ❋ *"I choose to believe I can do this."*
* ❋ *"I want this, and with practice I can do anything."*
* ❋ *"What I think about I bring about."*
* ❋ *"Today I am keeping my attention on my happiness and my health."*

*   *"I am powerful now, and I am accepting it."*
*   *"I take full responsibility for my body today."*
*   *"I care about how I feel, and I am ready to feel great."*

MIND/BODY EXERCISE:
BEGINNING THE PRACTICE

To open the IntenSati practice, we begin with a powerful warm-up for both your body and your mind:

> *"Every day in a very true way I co-create my reality.*
> *As above, so below. This is what I know."*

As you have learned in this chapter, every day you are creating your experience by the thoughts you choose to think, the perspective you choose to take, the attention you give to what you hate or what you love . . . or anything in between. You are always creating because you are always thinking.

Here is the important thing about your part in the co-creation process: You may not always have a say in your circumstances, but you always have a say in your *perspective* of the circumstances. You were born to the parents you were born to; you are as tall as you are going to be; you have a past you cannot change; you have the challenges you face. But either you can use those circumstances as proof of why you cannot be who you want to be, or you can see them as a starting point and go from there—you participate in the reality your life becomes. By choosing to accept where you are right now and dropping the complaining about it, you will create the opening for a new possibility, a new outcome, a new result!

The Sati life is a conscious, deliberate life. It's about loving, thriving, and taking the reins. Do this warm-up every day for thirty days. Write it down on a notecard and place it in many places that you can see throughout the day. Memorize it, say it over and over to yourself as you go about your day. Make it an imprint on your mind and your heart that *you* are the one responsible for your health and happiness. It takes just two minutes, and if you start every day with this declaration, you will awaken yourself to who you really are. No longer will you see yourself as powerless, unworthy, or unable. Instead, you will begin to see that great things are within your grasp.

Before you begin, stand in the ready pose, hands at your heart, eyes closed, and repeat to yourself your intention: "I intend to feel good" or "I intend to feel better." You are warming up your body and your mind together. Once you learn the entire exercise outlined here, do it for at least two minutes. You are harnessing your power of concentration. Even though you may feel that you are "just thinking it," try not to let your mind wander.

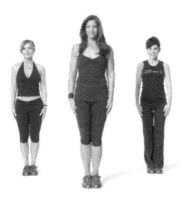

READY: Stand tall, your eyes straight ahead, feet together, and shoulders back, with your arms by your sides. This pose represents your readiness to take action now.

FIRST-ROUND ACTION

Hold each action while repeating the affirmation below.

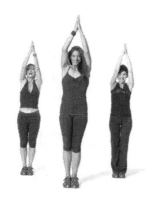

RESPONSIBILITY FOR LIFE: Standing tall with your feet together, raise your arms over your head, press your palms together in the pose of Responsibility, and silently say, *"With gratitude, I take full responsibility for my health and happiness."*

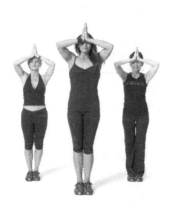

RESPONSIBILITY FOR MIND: With your palms still pressed together, bring your hands to the center of your forehead, your third eye of inner wisdom, to the pose of Will and silently say, *"With gratitude, I take full responsibility for the power of my thoughts."*

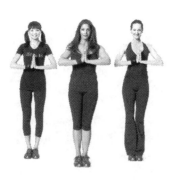

RESPONSIBILITY FOR ATTITUDE: Bring your hands to your heart and silently say, *"With gratitude, I take full responsibility for the power of my emotions."*

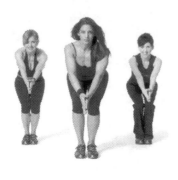

RESPONSIBILITY FOR AC-TIONS: Bend your knees to a chair pose, keeping your legs together, as if you are sitting in a chair. With your palms pressed together, extend your arms from your heart toward the floor (make sure to keep your back straight), and silently say, *"With gratitude, I take full responsibility for the power of my actions."*

SECOND-ROUND ATTITUDE

Repeat the actions, and this time feel the gratitude begin to awaken within you with this new perspective. Inhale as you extend up and exhale as you extend down.

RHYTHM OF THE ACTIONS: Arms up for 2 counts. Single counts: forehead—heart—floor.

Silently say, "Up for two, forehead, heart, floor."

THIRD-ROUND AFFIRMATION, PART 1

Now do the same actions twice, this time reciting this affirmation out loud:

As the arms extend overhead to the pose of Responsibility, say, "Every day" for 2 counts.

As your arms come down to your forehead, heart, and floor say,
 "In a very" (single count forehead)

"true" (single count heart)
"way" (single count floor)

As your arms go up a second time, say, "I cocreate" (2 counts).

As your arms go down a second time to the forehead, heart, and floor, say, "My Reality."
"My" (single count forehead)
"reality" (single count heart)
Pause (single count floor)

Repeat from the top.

"Every day in a very true way I cocreate my reality" (repeat for one minute).

THIRD-ROUND AFFIRMATION, PART 2

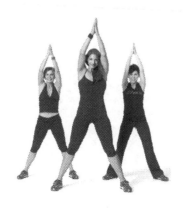
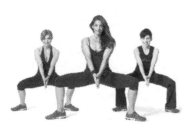

RESPONSIBILITY:

Stand with your feet more than shoulder width apart, slightly turned out, with straight legs. Your arms are straight over your head, your palms touching in the pose of Responsibility.

Bend your knees so your thighs are parallel to the floor and your knees are over your ankles (not over your toes). Make sure to keep your back straight and your abs in. Extend your arms straight down, with your palms together in front of your body.

Repeat the action and move your body with the attitude of gratitude for what you are able to do. Inhale as your arms go up and
exhale as they come down.

RHYTHM OF THE ACTIONS: Arms up for 2 counts / Arms
down for 2 counts / Arms up and down for 4 single counts.

Say, "Up for two, down for two, four singles."

As your arms go up for 2 counts, say, "As above."

As you arms come down and you bend your knees for 2 counts,
say, "So below."

As your arms go up and down on single counts, say, "This—is—
what I—know."

Repeat for one minute.

Now put parts 1 and 2 together.

WARRIOR / READY

"ARE YOU A WARRIOR?"

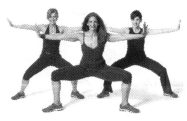

WARRIOR: Take a wide V-stance, turn out your feet, and bend your knees, making sure to keep your knees in line with your ankles. Pull up from your center with a tall spine, straighten your arms out to either side of your body, and flex your wrists.

"AND ARE YOU READY?"

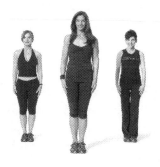

READY: Stand tall, your eyes straight ahead, feet together, and shoulders back, with your arms by your sides. This pose represents your readiness to take action now.

Stand with your feet together, eyes closed, one hand over your heart. Take a deep breath in and bring your intention back to your mind.

CHAPTER CHECKLIST
i Will . . .

* Take 100 percent responsibility for living a life I love in a body I love.

* Strive to change my negative thoughts to positive ones.

* Write the IntenSati warm-up on a notecard or Post-it and place it in my home or office. I will start every morning saying it as I prepare for the day.

principle two

DESIRE IS THE FIRE FOR CHANGING YOUR LIFE

---

o you want it? No, do you really, *really* want it?

You may think, "Patricia, what a dumb question! Who doesn't want to be thinner, fitter, happier, and healthier? Of course I want it."

Well, wanting it is one thing; *desiring* it—putting passion to that want and fueling that want with 100 percent of your mind, body, and soul—is another. Desire is the fire of transformation. When you really, *really* want something, you must keep your attention focused on the joy of achieving it instead of the pain of not having it, and you will succeed. This change in focus is the cornerstone of succeeding in your new, healthy life. Nothing can derail you or distract you from your goal when you focus on joy. You have to see what you want—to feel stronger, healthier, and calmer, and to look better—then wrap your arms, your heart, and your mind around that vision and refuse to let go. I believe that you want it; now *you* have to believe it.

Desire is all-powerful; it can give you courage where there was paralyzing fear, superhuman strength where there was once weakness. It is the same energy that helps a mother lift a car off her child, when in normal circumstances she would never be able to do it. All you need to do to tap into your desire is to take your attention off where you are and where you have been and firmly place it on where you want to go. But often, we are unwilling to truly allow ourselves to feel the deep desire of wanting something because we fear not getting it or achieving it. How often have you muted your desire for something because you were afraid of disappointment? Declaring what you want takes tremendous courage! Desire is not about wishing it will happen; it's not saying, "Patricia, I want to fit into my skinny jeans" or "I want to swim a mile." It's about taking responsibility to allow it to happen. It's resisting that candy bar at the vending machine or walking home instead of taking the bus because doing these things proves your commitment to improving your body and your life.

As you learned in Principle 1, change starts with your inner dialogue. Are you focusing on the pain of being where you are rather than the process of getting where you want to be? To reverse your focus, you need to get in touch with what you really want, who you want to be, how you want to live, and what is really important to you. Do any of the following statements sound like something you might be thinking? Many times the "but" word is your red flag that you are derailing your own desire:

> "I really want to lose weight, **but** my metabolism is so slow."
> "I really want to be thinner, **but** everyone in my family is overweight."
> "I really want to go to the gym, **but** I am so embarrassed by how I look."
> "I really want to lose weight, **but** it's so hard and I don't have time."

Not one of these statements is empowering, and none of them activates your personal fire of desire. They are conflicting, confusing, and just a bunch of excuses. You don't need excuses. Either choose to really change your body, your health, and your life and go for it, or take it off your list of desires. Stop talking about how much you hate your body, and give your powerful attention to something else, something you really want.

Desire is your call to action: "I am ready. I am willing. I can do it." You will consciously and deliberately use the power of the passion that is ignited within you when you see yourself at the finish line. Take your attention off all the difficulties you might face and the discomforts you might endure, and let the vision of your success fill your mind and your heart.

Take Each Day One Moment at a Time

This principle of desire is about becoming clear about what you want: every day your desire helps you make better choices for yourself. Each time you are confronted with a choice you must make, summon your inner warrior—the one that is telling you, "You are worthy of the life you envision! Go ahead! Make it happen!" See your goal; see your future; see the person you desire to be. Now see the choice before you: What should you order for lunch, a salad with grilled chicken or a bacon double cheeseburger? What would the new you—not the old you—do? This is not just willpower at work; it's your desire fueling your plan. And when you make the right choice, something inside you will sing. You will feel the difference. Notice it; give yourself a pat on the back for it, and know that each positive choice you make is a rung on the ladder. From here on, the climb gets easier and easier.

This is a mind game, and to help you make the best choices for yourself, you must see throughout the day the new way of life

CONNECTING TO YOUR DESIRE:
A WRITING EXERCISE

Sit down for five minutes with a pen and blank sheet of paper before you. Our goal is for you not to just write a list of what you want to do; it's to help you realize *why* you want it.

At the top of the sheet, write "I want . . ." and fill it in with words that articulate what you want.

Now, beneath it, write the following: "I intend to achieve this because . . ."

Allow yourself to fill the paper with any positive thoughts that come to mind: *"I intend to achieve this because . . . I deserve it. I am ready for it. I am strong, smart, a good wife, a good mom, a kind friend. I deserve to be healthy, happy, and proud, and I am tired of not feeling that way. It's my turn. It's my time. I can do this. I will do this . . ."*

Just write nonstop. Even if you repeat things over and over, or the words don't make total sense, just let the ideas flow. You may want to play a song that inspires you in the background, as music helps activate emotions.

Now read your words. Contemplate them. Visualize them. What do they tell you about yourself? Where do they point you? How do they ring in your ears? How do they make you feel? Look for your motivation and use your words to clarify what it is you really want versus what you are afraid of, or don't want. If you are ever struggling to connect with your desire, go back and reread these words. Let them lift you, inspire you, energize you. These words come from your heart and can empower you. 🔲

you want to have. Something inside of you is urging you, begging you, encouraging you to try something new: to do what will feel better, to make a choice that will empower you to feel good and be happy. So when I ask you now, "Do you want it?" dig down deep and find your inner truth and desire. Close your eyes;

see your future in your grasp. Don't be afraid. Don't worry about the long term or the how. For right now, just reignite the wanting, the desire, and the fire of transformation within you. You're ready for action! Bring it on!

The Whiner vs. the Warrior

I have discovered that there are really only two types of people in life: the whiners and the warriors. The whiners keep resisting change; they're afraid that they won't make it. The fear of another failure is too great. But the warriors turn their attention to the goal and the future vision; their eyes are constantly on the prize.

I want you to listen to the voice of the whiner. What does it sound like? Meek, pained, powerless: "But *why* can't I have it? *Why* me? Woe is me!" It's the voice of guilt, resentment, weakness. The whiner mind-set is one of defeat before the journey even begins.

The warrior mind-set is certain of victory and willing to face the challenge, the discomfort, and the obstacles. The warrior has his mind firmly placed on the goal. She chooses perseverance, integrity, and courage. She says, "Yes, I want it! I don't mind giving this up to get where I want to be!" Hers is the voice of power, triumph, and spirit.

Which voice is yours?

> ### Words to live by
>
> *What I resist will persist.*
>
> *Today I choose to go with the flow.*
>
> *I now believe I will succeed!*
>
> *My desire is strong, and that's enough.*
>
> *I'm confident now, and I will allow all good to come to me.*
>
> *When I lighten up, I am movin' on up!*
>
> *I become who I am meant to be.*

Take a moment and write down all your complaints, your reasons and excuses for why you can't lose weight, why you can't feel better, why you never get it "right." Now, step back and take a good look at what you've written. What will be magnificently obvious to you is *why* you remain where you are. Up until now, you haven't chosen a new dialogue or a new script. The whiner in winning! Here are some of my favorites:

I don't have time.
I have tried before.
I hate healthy food.
I have no willpower.
I hate skinny people.
I come from fat genes.
I have no discipline.
I don't know how to cook.
I am too hungry all the time.
I don't care about how I look or feel.
I've given up.
I am afraid if I lose weight I still won't be happy . . . so why try?
I could never give up my favorite foods.
I hate to be hungry.
I can't do it.

The whiner has a lot of power, and unless you deactivate him, he will run the show forever. A warrior, on the other hand, is someone who stands for living a life she loves in a body she loves. Here are some of my favorite warrior cries:

I believe in myself.
I believe I will succeed.
I am ready to change.
I am willing to change.

I am able to change.
I am changing right now!
I can do it!

Pick any one of these lines and repeat it over and over to yourself. Make one (or several) your warrior mantra. It will get stuck in your head (since you can think only one way at a time), and you will be living and breathing the warrior mentality. Think of this statement as the guardian angel of your body.

Creating a Vision Board

Vision boards put a face on your desire and remind you of your new vision of yourself. Take a posterboard or corkboard and begin to fill it up. Go through magazines and cut out pictures of whatever inspires and motivates you: body parts you admire, places you want to go, foods you want to enjoy. Add quotes, affirmations, and pictures of people who support you and inspire you, who have transformed themselves, too. Write notes to yourself, like "Yes, you can!" or "Yes, I want this! Obstacles? So what! I will do it anyway!" You can either sit down and do it all at once or look daily for things to hang up on your board and keep adding as you go along.

Make sure to put your vision board somewhere you will see it. Look at it first thing in the morning and last thing at night. And every time you look at it, just imagine yourself *there* for a moment. Feel the dream growing, the vision getting stronger, the inspiration in you gaining momentum. Every time you pause and feel it, you are fueling that incredible fire within you. And when that passion is palpable, nothing will stand in your way!

The Words of the Warrior

This is the warrior declaration. Say it every morning, not just as a prayer or a wish but as a command to yourself.

Today I stand as a warrior and I choose to be all I can be.

I stand for excellence in all areas of my life.

I am dedicated to an extraordinary degree to loving my life and living my life's calling.

I choose perseverance, courage, integrity, and impeccability.

I look for confidence and approval in my own heart and mind, and what others think of me makes no difference.

I know that it is ultimately how I feel about myself that gives me the experience of my life, and that shame, guilt, regret, and resentment are the most deadly of all opponents. The only way they can be defeated is by absolute integrity, or the absence of contradiction between what I know, what I profess, and what I do.

I know that when I lie to myself I am severed from my truth, which is my power, and an inharmonious relationship to my truth is deadly.

No one is born a warrior, just as no one is born average. We make ourselves that way by the accumulation of steps we take toward one or the other.

I know the power of my mind, and I begin every journey confident of victory. I am defeated only when I have accepted defeat. The moment I turn my back on myself and my vision may be the moment I halt just short of my goal, making all my previous efforts useless.

My work is to discover my work and with all my heart give myself to it, and by honoring this path, I will achieve the greatest victory of all: a life of love, a life I love, and a life well lived.

Today I choose the path of the warrior.

IGNITE YOUR DESIRE

Yes, I have a dream.
This time is mine.
I am free
to declare
my destiny.

Do each move for at least one minute before going on to the next move. You should feel your heart rate increase and your muscles burning a bit before you stop (ideally, 20 minutes, so you can get the maximum benefit). If it is easy for you to speak and move at the same time, increase the energy of the action. If you are not able to speak out loud, decrease the energy in the action. The goal is to learn the moves and to link the words and the actions together, so you can move into the cardio, endorphin-releasing phase.

Feel what you are saying! Embody these phrases. Hold your dream in your mind, and know that when you are thinking about your goals with enthusiasm, you are declaring your destiny!

COMMITMENT

SAY, "YES!"

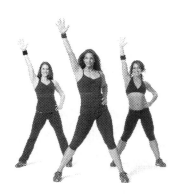

Stand with your feet more than shoulder width apart. Reach your right arm straight up over your head while slightly bending your right knee. Keep your left arm bent at your side. Both palms are facing forward.

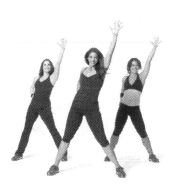

Now switch your arms, reaching your left arm straight up over your head while slightly bending your left knee. Keep your right arm bent by your side. Both palms are facing forward.

FOCUS

SAY, "I HAVE A DREAM."

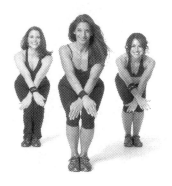

Keeping both arms straight and your palms down, cross your arms in front of you in a slicing motion as you bend your knees deeply.

VICTORY

SAY, "THIS TIME IS MINE."

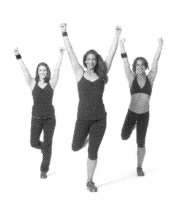

Fully extend your arms over your head, making a V for victory as you jog in place.

HAPPY

SAY, "I AM FREE"

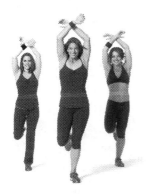

Keep your legs together and your back straight as you bend your knees. Extend your arms and cross them in front of you.

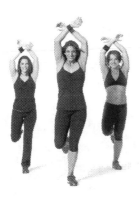

As you jump into the air, circle your arms away from you in giant sweeping arcs.

WILLPOWER

SAY, "TO DECLARE"

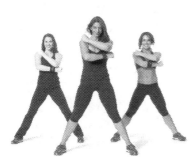

Your legs are straight in a wide V-stance; make sure to keep your knees over your ankles, and keep your back straight and your abs in. With your hands in fists and your elbows bent in front of you, roll your arms *away* from your body as fast as you can, going into a deep knee bend.

ACCEPTANCE

SAY, "MY DESTINY."

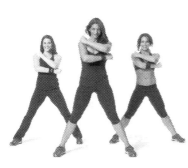

Your legs are straight in a wide V-stance, with your hands in fists and your elbows bent in front of you. Roll your arms toward your body as fast as you can. Stand straight and jog in place. Keeping your hands in fists and your elbows still bent, this time roll your arms *toward* you as fast as you can, raising your elbows to the sky. Now reverse the direction, rolling your arms away from you.

MY SATI LIFE READING LIST

I read books often to help me remember my truth and my purpose and to uplift my spirit in times when I feel down. One of my favorite daily activities is to just pick up a book and open it to any page and see perfection. I urge you to read books that encourage you and raise you up. Each of these books made a deep impression on me and my view of myself:

❊ *Happiness NOW!* by Robert Holden

❊ *Power vs. Force* by David R. Hawkins

❊ *Ask and It Is Given* by Esther and Jerry Hicks

❊ *Tao Te Ching* by Guy Leekley

❊ *The Greatest Salesman in the World* by Og Mandino

❊ *Molecules of Emotion* by Candace B. Pert, Ph.D.

❊ *Think and Grow Rich* by Napoleon Hill

❊ *The Law of Success* by Napoleon Hill

❊ *The Power of Awareness* by Neville Goddard

❊ *The Power of Intention* by Dr. Wayne Dyer

SERIES BREAKDOWN

After you have done each exercise for at least one minute, it's time to break down the series and run it through.

Say, "Yes! I have a dream," for 1 to 2 minutes.
- "Yes!" is the pose of COMMITMENT. Alternate your arms overhead for 4 counts.
- "I have a dream" is FOCUS. Slice your arms in front of you for 4 counts.

Say, "This time is mine. I am free," for 1 to 2 minutes.
- "This time is mine" is VICTORY. Extend arms overhead in a V and jog in place for 4 counts.
- "I am free" is HAPPY. Jump and sweep your arms away from you two times in 4 counts.

Now run through from the top for 1 to 2 minutes.
- "Yes"—COMMITMENT—4 counts
- "I have a dream"—FOCUS—4 counts
- "This time is mine"—VICTORY—4 counts
- "I am free"—HAPPY—4 counts

Say, "To declare my destiny" for 1 to 2 minutes.
- "To declare" is WILLPOWER. Roll your arms *away* from you for 4 counts.
- "My destiny" is ACCEPTANCE. Roll your arms *toward* you for 4 counts.

Now run through from the top for 1 to 2 minutes.
- "Yes!"—COMMITMENT—4 counts
- "I have a dream"—FOCUS—4 counts
- "This time is mine"—VICTORY—4 counts
- "I am free"—HAPPY—4 counts
- "To declare"—WILLPOWER—4 counts
- "My destiny"—ACCEPTANCE—4 counts

CHAPTER CHECKLIST
i will . . .

* Keep my attention on what I want. I will write down my goal as if it were already achieved. For example, "I am now 125 pounds and I love it!"

* Every time I feel tempted to take an action that goes against my goal, stop and ask myself, "Am I being a warrior or a whiner?"

* Make a vision board and put it somewhere where I can see it often.

principle three

ALL YOU ARE—AND ALL YOU WILL BE—IS A RESULT OF HOW DEEPLY YOU HONOR YOURSELF

I had a student once—let's call her Mary—who said to me, "Patricia, I would give my right arm to be able to lose forty pounds." I replied, "Well, all you really have to give up is a few extra calories and you can keep your right arm."

It doesn't have to be that hard to drop weight, certainly not worth losing a limb over! It's pretty black and white: drop the drama, eat less, move more, and care about how you feel in your own skin. But it's easier to believe it *is* hard, even impossible, and that the fates are conspiring against you. Of course, Mary didn't mean she would *really* give her right arm. But the message she was sending me (and herself) was that her weight was not where she would like it to be and that it wasn't her fault. There was nothing she could do; she was dealt a bum hand, and this was the life she had ended up living.

I have news for Mary, and for you, too, if you wake up most days feeling "Woe is me!" Things are not out of your hands or your control. You are writing your story, moment by moment, thought by thought, and your body and your life are only a reflection and a consequence of what you are choosing. Think about this: What happens when you remove the drama, the lack of responsibility, and the victim mentality from your life? What do you have left? You and your choices.

You may not think that you choose obesity, heart disease, joint pain, hypertension, stroke, cardiovascular disease, congestive heart failure, fatty liver disease, gout, or sleep apnea—to name a few ailments. But if you are not choosing health, you are choosing illness. What you eat, how you live, how often you exercise, the stress you endure, the amount of sleep you get, how much alcohol you drink, and how much you smoke are all choices you make. If you believe that your body and your health are out of your control, then you choose to give up your power and your peace of mind.

All the tools have been handed to you to create the experience of your life. You've been given the responsibility of using these tools mindfully, with awareness and with intention. Are you honoring this privilege by creating the health and wellness you deserve? When you get a result that is not what you want, use it as an opportunity to stop, pay attention, and bring more awareness to the way you are living. Ask yourself, "What can I do *right now* to feel even a little better?" Then "Am I willing to do that?" You have the power; you have the desire; but are you honoring your intentions every day in every way? Or are you sabotaging your efforts by not believing you are worthy or capable of what you want to be?

There is no amount of action or "doing" that can take the place of honoring yourself. When it comes to the care of your body, it doesn't end when you reach your goal weight. It is a daily commitment to your happiness. The bottom line is that every choice you make comes from either love or fear. When your choices come from fear, they will lead you to more suffering;

PATRICIA MORENO

when your choices come from love, they will connect you to the happiness that has been within you all along. You just couldn't feel it because you can't feel fear and love at the same time; you have to choose. You *can* choose.

A New Way to Cope with Conflict

We all contend with pain, sorrow, or disappointment at one time or another. It's part of life. Frankly, you'd never know what happiness is unless you experienced the other side of the coin. Part of honoring yourself is not running away from these emotions. These feelings—as excruciating as they may seem at the time—are there for a reason. When they come up, I'd like you to do this: Stop, feel them, wonder why they're there, and recognize that they can guide you back on track. Resist the urge to run away from the bad feelings. Awareness gives you the opportunity to see the bigger picture and to bring love and honor back to yourself.

For example, you wake up one morning and you have *had* it. You're tired of being tired and fed up with complaining about how you look and feel. You're tired of not doing anything about it. So you get your diet book and you make a plan to start *today*. You get past Days 1, 2, 3, and maybe even 4, but then something happens: You have a bad day at work or a fight with your husband, or a bill comes in the mail. Whatever the situation, you now feel uneasy, tense, hurt, unhappy. You think, "I deserve a break!" and you can practically hear that pint of ice cream in the freezer beckoning.

You're right; you *do* deserve a break. But does a break really come in the form of ice cream, a brownie, or a bag of chips? Taking a positive step instead—by making a good food choice or working out—will help you handle this tough time, and the ones that will inevitably come up later. Instead of compounding the problem, you will be compounding the commitment.

Instead of reaching for that brownie, I want you to do the following:

1. Stop!

2. Feel the emotion or stress.

3. Realize that you can do something to make yourself feel better.

4. Remember your commitment to yourself.

5. Realize that a "quick fix" isn't going to solve your other problems.

6. Honor the privilege you have to choose a new path: make a healthy food choice, work out, meditate, etc.

The Lies We Tell Ourselves

I was at my thinnest weight, 140 pounds, in 1991, when I was participating in the National Aerobics Championships and had been training and dieting hard. It was my biggest fear to be on that stage and to lose because I was too fat. I was horrified that this would happen and was actually almost certain it would. I was in a panic. Even though at five feet, ten inches with a large frame I was lean and muscular, I felt I would never be thin enough and would *never* be able to maintain this weight.

I had gotten to this weight by bingeing and purging and also overexercising. Yes, it had worked, but I could never keep it up—and that added to my shame and self-loathing. Here I was, thin, yet all I could think was how miserable and embarrassed I was going to be when I gained it all back. And even though from the outside it looked as if I were displaying great amounts of courage, discipline, and strength, on the inside I felt the worst I had ever felt.

Where was the joy and happiness I was supposed to be experiencing at this point in my life? I couldn't enjoy my successes because I never believed in myself. I never believed this champion athlete was who I was. I felt like a fake, a phony, a farce. The entire time it was as if I were masquerading. I wasn't this thin aerobics champ; I was really a lazy, chubby girl, with no discipline or willpower. You see, I was trying to change from the outside, but my belief never changed. You can guess what happened: I gained the weight right back, and I fell deeper and deeper into despair.

> ## Words to live by
>
> *Doubt your doubts and they vanish!*
>
> *Feel your fears and they fade!*
>
> *Let go of your worries and they will let go of you!*
>
> *Honor and respect yourself, live up to your personal standards.*
>
> *Give all of yourself and you will have all!*

Only when I acknowledged how I was feeling could I start to see the truth. I was hurting my body, not honoring it. And when I started to dig deeper, to let the true feelings bubble to the surface instead of burying them, those deep fears and secrets that I was afraid to face or feel turned out to be the very emotions that woke me up. When I realized I had had enough of the darkness, I started reaching for the light. I took my attention off of thinness as the goal and put happiness and freedom on my priority list. Let this be your guide: The truth feels good, lies don't.

When Other People Are the Problem

Unfortunately, there are many people who make living a healthier lifestyle hard for you. Maybe it's your kids, who eat all the junky food you can't. Or the family members always trying to feed you ("Eat! Eat! I made it especially for you!"). Or your girl-friends who want to go out for drinks instead of going to the gym. Or maybe it's your husband, boyfriend, or even BFF, who fears that if you lose weight and change, you won't want him anymore. "You're on *another* diet?" he asks disapprovingly. Other people's fear can be your worst enemy.

What should you do, lose their phone numbers? Ask your kids to eat their Oreos out of your sight? Tell your buddies that you can't go out for cosmos *ever*? None of the above. Who is in control here, you or them? Whose life is it? Whose body is it? You make the decisions; you call the shots. And if you are honoring your commitment to yourself, others will see it and feel it and you will find a way to make it work. Ask yourself this: Are you using these "derailers" as a good excuse to let yourself off the hook? You're not a victim unless you allow yourself to be one.

I get it. Sometimes it's just easier to say, "Well, I *had* to go out for a business dinner last night . . ." as if that's a good excuse for why you overate and drank and skipped your spin class this morning. No one said it was going to be easy to make the changes you want to make. But if you are firm in your desire and you act like it, then other people can't knock you down. You also have to give people direction: You have to say what you need, ask for support, just say no, find new friends, feed your children well, and plan your day.

When you honor yourself and fit everything else in around you, others will respond to what you're putting out there. They'll become your supporting cast and crew. Your commitment has to be rock-solid. A light gust of wind shouldn't come along and blow away your goal. If you really want to make your life easier, then make gym friends, get workout partners, put your family on the plan, or arrange business meetings at places you know have something on the menu that fits into your lifestyle. Have the world work around you and for you.

The novelist/lyricist Paulo Coelho said, "When you want something, all the universe conspires in helping you to achieve it." When you honor yourself and your happiness as your best and most important priority, people see you how you see yourself. If you are honoring yourself, respecting yourself, caring about yourself, others will, too. And even if some don't, it won't matter. Ultimately, it's a question of your commitment to your happiness, health, and peace of mind. Build your belief in yourself that you are worth it, you deserve it, you come first, and your happiness is what your loved ones want for you. You can have it all . . . but you have to take it, own it, ask for it, and mean it!

Ways to Honor Yourself

I want you to make it your goal to honor yourself in some small way, each and every day. Never feel guilty for being good to yourself, and never neglect giving attention to your desire. These little tasks and treats will remind you of your goal and your greatness! Choose at least one a day, but feel free to schedule in several.

* Start your day off with an affirmation that gets you going in the right direction—one that reminds you to be who you want to be.
* Eat well.
* Work out.
* Go for a walk.
* Sit still and do nothing for five minutes.
* Read a good book.
* Call a friend.
* Get a manicure.
* Get a massage.
* List all the things you are avoiding, and make a plan to deal with them.

* Clean your home; get rid of things you don't need anymore, and clean out the clutter.
* Get a haircut.
* Buy some fresh flowers.
* Weigh yourself instead of avoiding the truth.
* Tell the truth.
* Make new friends.
* Speak your opinion.
* Trust yourself.
* Listen to your heart.
* Go to bed early.
* Get up an hour earlier so you don't have to rush.
* Have some fun.
* Go on a vacation.
* Get a better job or ask for a raise.
* Say a prayer.
* Listen to some soothing music.
* Dance out your stress.
* Take a nap.
* Meditate.
* Snuggle with someone or a pet.
* Open the windows and let in the fresh air.
* Smile, laugh, cry.
* Draw, paint, or build something.
* Work on your vision board.
* Breathe . . . just breathe.

Say It with Me . . .

Start your day with a few affirmations. Here are some of my favorites to help you channel the strength you need to relinquish the past:

* *I am accepting now.*
* *I am free now.*
* *I am the peace I want to see.*
* *I surrender the past and step forward confidently.*
* *All I need is within me now, for my life, all others, and myself.*
* *I accept I have the power to choose to drop the old for the new.*
* *I am worth it today, and I am taking action.*

MIND/BODY EXERCISE:
I AM WILLING TO BE IT!

I know where I want to go.
I know who I have to be.
I am willing to be it.
I will take this opportunity.
I believe I will succeed!

Do each move for at least one minute before going on to the next move. You should feel your heart rate increase and your muscles burning a bit before you stop (ideally, 20 minutes, so you can get the maximum benefit).

These exercises are all about taking action. If you don't take action, you are just a dreamer! They will increase your heart rate, and you will also feel your hamstrings and buttocks burning. That's a good sign—keep it up!

ABLE

SAY, "I KNOW WHERE I WANT TO GO."

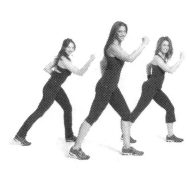

Pivot to the left and take a runner's stance, as if you were just about to take off in a sprint. Slightly bend your left knee, keeping your left foot flat on the floor and your right heel raised. Your elbows are bent, with your right arm in front of your body and your left arm behind you.

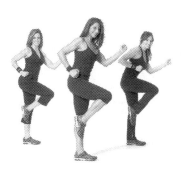

Like a spring, straighten your left leg and bring your right foot to meet the left knee. Switch your arm position as your knee comes up. Really feel like you are taking off.

READY TO TAKE ACTION

SAY, "I KNOW WHO I HAVE TO BE."

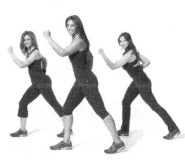

Now pivot to the right and take a runner's stance on the opposite side. Slightly bend your right knee, keeping your right foot flat on the floor and your left heel raised. Your elbows are slightly bent, with your left arm in front of your body and your right arm behind you.

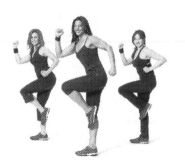

Just as on the other side, energetically straighten your right leg and bring your left foot up to meet your right knee. Again, switch your arm position as your knee comes up.

WILLING

SAY, "I AM WILLING TO BE IT."

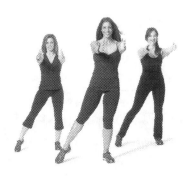

Stand on your left leg, knee slightly bent. Point your right foot out from your right side and touch the floor with your toes. Extend your arms parallel to the floor in front of you, shoulder width apart, with your palms facing.

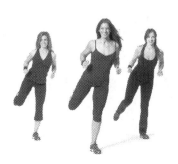

Bend your right knee behind you and kick your butt with your heel. At the same time, slice your arms down by your sides with your elbows bent.

Give yourself a kick in the behind to remind yourself to drop the whining and complaining and just get into action and do what you can do now! Try to touch your heel to your buttocks every time. If you can't reach the first time, keep trying.

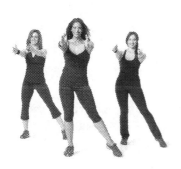

Now step your right foot down, and point your left foot directly to the side and touch the floor with your left toe. Once again, extend the arms parallel to the floor and shoulder width apart with your palms facing.

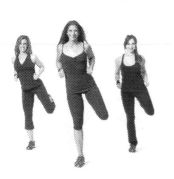

Repeating the same move on the other side, bend your left knee behind you and kick your butt with your heel. At the same time, slice your arms down by your sides with your elbows bent.

DESIRE

SAY, "I WILL TAKE THIS OPPORTUNITY."

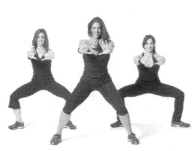

Assume the Warrior stance. Your hands are in front of you, with your thumbs and index fingers touching to create a triangle in front of your heart. Remain in the Warrior stance. Keeping the triangle sign with your hands, passionately extend your arms from your heart center.

The more you bend your knees, the more challenging the move will be, and the more you extend your arms and keep the enthusiasm up, the more you will link the action and the affirmation, making it a powerful life- and body-altering duo!

FAITH

SAY, "I BELIEVE I WILL SUCCEED!"

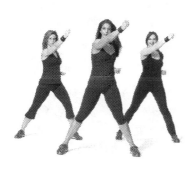

Stand with your feet hip width apart. Bend your elbows with your fists at either side of your chin. Powerfully punch your right fist up and diagonally across your body, allowing your torso to rotate to the left.

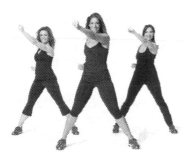

Bring your right fist back beside your chin and now powerfully punch your left fist up and diagonally across your body, allowing your torso to rotate to the right. Keep your elbows close to your side and bring both fists back to either side of your chin after each punch.

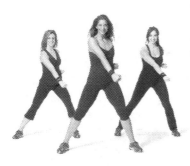

With your knees bent, powerfully punch your right fist down and diagonally across your body, allowing your torso to rotate to the left. Make sure to keep your back straight and your abs in as you punch down.

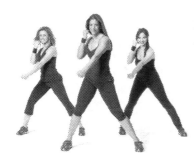

Bring your right fist back beside your chin and now powerfully punch your left fist down and diagonally across your body, allowing your torso to rotate to the right.

Remember to keep your elbows close to your sides and bring both fists back to either side of your chin after each punch!

SERIES BREAKDOWN

After you have done each exercise for at least one minute, it's time to break down the series and run it through.

Say, "I know where I want to go, I know who I have to be, I am willing to be it."

"I know where I want to go"—READY TO TAKE ACTION. Pivot left and lift the right knee up and down four times for 8 counts.

- "I know" (knee up and down for 2 counts)
- "where" (knee up and down for 2 counts)
- "I want" (knee up and down for 2 counts)
- "to go" (knee up and down for 2 counts)

"I know who I have to be"—READY TO TAKE ACTION. Pivot right and lift the left knee up four times for 8 counts.

- "I know" (knee up and down for 2 counts)
- "who" (knee up and down for 2 counts)
- "I have" (knee up and down for 2 counts)
- "to be" (knee up and down for 2 counts)

"I am willing to be it"—WILLING. Alternate kicking each heel to your butt for 8 counts.

- "I" (kick butt 2 counts)
- "am" (knee up and down for 2 counts)
- "willing to be" (knee up and down for 2 counts)
- "it" (knee up and down for 2 counts)

Run through the entire phrase for one to two minutes.

- "I know where I want to go"—ABLE (8 counts)
- "I know who I have to be"—READY TO TAKE ACTION (8 counts)
- "I am willing to be it"—WILLING (8 counts)

Say, "I will take this opportunity. I believe I will succeed."

"I will take this opportunity"—DESIRE. Extend arms in and out, hands in a triangle position, for 8 counts.
- "I"—2 counts
- "will take"—2 counts
- "this opportunity"—4 counts

"I believe I will succeed"—FAITH. Alternate punching arms up/up and down/down, for 8 counts.
- "I"—punch up right and left for 2 counts
- "believe"—punch down right and left for 2 counts
- "I will"—punch up right and left for 2 counts
- "succeed"—punch up right and left for 2 counts

Now run through from the top for one to two minutes:
- "I know where I want to go"—ABLE (8 counts)
- "I know who I have to be"—READY TO TAKE ACTION (8 counts)
- "I am willing to be it"—WILLING (8 counts)
- "I will take this opportunity"—DESIRE (8 counts)
- "I believe I will succeed"—FAITH (8 counts)

CHAPTER CHECKLIST

i will . . .

✳ Listen to myself . . . and not be swayed by others' negativity or doubt.

✳ Make time for me. I will honor my intentions by making myself a priority.

✳ Try not to react to conflict/stress with actions (such as overeating) that go against my goals.

principle four

PRACTICE WHAT YOU PREACH: EMBODY YOUR AFFIRMATIONS

*W*here does your mind go when you are working out? Are you zoning out watching TV? Are you reading some article in a magazine or blasting music on your MP3 player? Or maybe you're just staring at the timer on the treadmill thinking, "I have to do this for ten more minutes? I am going to die!"

Guilty as charged? We all are. Sometimes you are mentally engaged and motivated, and other times you are complaining and whining or simply spacing out. But I will let you in on a little secret: the more engaged you are in your workout and the more focused, the longer and harder you will be able to work out. The reason the IntenSati workout is so effective in helping people transform their lives is that it is action with integrity. You are literally practicing *being* who you want to be. You are training yourself to speak, act, and think like a warrior and a winner!

Through this program, you practice being, speaking, thinking, and acting more positively, more courageously, more lovingly, and more compassionately all at once. You train yourself mentally, emotionally, and physically. You build your awareness of yourself and experience in the present moment the results of declaring positive statements such as "Yes! I am committed!" "Yes! I have willpower! I have the strength!" "Every single day I am better and better in every way!"

Here's what it boils down to: You can practice being who you want to be. You have been practicing "being you" all your life. Now, by putting the exercise portion of this program into action, you will practice being enthusiastic, committed, courageous, deliberate. You are fully engaged, and watching TV while working out will feel like a distraction. You won't need it. We usually want to distract ourselves from our complaining. But now, all your attention is focused on those positive emotions that will fuel your workout.

If you are enthusiastic about what you are doing—engaged, passionate, determined, committed, willing, and accepting—regardless of what it is, you perform much better. And not only are the results better, but your enjoyment of the activity is heightened. When you are feeling good while you are doing something, it reinforces your desire to do it again. Think about the things you enjoy doing and how much more likely you are to work them into your schedule.

Or think of something you have been successful in during the course of your life: You won that spelling bee in grade school! You graduated college summa cum laude! You landed that promotion at work! In each case, what was your mental attitude toward this challenge? Were you committed to and focused on it—or tuned out? Get the picture? Focusing this kind of attention and enthusiasm on your diet and fitness will reshape your ability to maintain your weight and health—no more yo-yoing, no more fads.

Giving Voice to Action

Inspired action is action you are taking *willingly*. When you are acting unwillingly, it is like going downhill with the brakes on. If you just take your foot off the brakes, stop the complaining, actually hold empowering thoughts, and find something to appreciate in the action, you will be speeding down that hill in record time with tremendous ease—and the time spent will be more enjoyable. Your goal in this chapter is to find the presence of joy, desire, and integrity in every move you make.

When I first started teaching this workout program, many people were resistant to speaking the positive statements out loud. It was different. No one was teaching this kind of workout, and I had a ton of skeptics who told me they felt silly, self-conscious, and awkward shouting to the heavens. Some were even annoyed at all the positivity in the room! "Does there have to be so much talking? Can't we just work out?" In a room of sixty people, I began with one or two who were daring enough to shout out loud.

After about six months, the classes continued to be packed, yet still fewer than a third of the people were willing to vocalize the statements. I came into class one day and had a heart-to-heart with my group. I told them, "From now on, if you are not willing to participate fully in this class the way it is designed, I am going to ask you to take another class. There are plenty of other classes for you that are good workouts. I am teaching something new. I am teaching about the power of how you think, and how when you think and speak a powerful statement while taking powerful action, the results will be powerful. Those of you not interested are in the wrong class!" I went on to suggest that if they were even willing to hold the thoughts *mentally* without saying them out loud at first, they would feel the powerful impact of congruent action.

Well, I don't know if it was that suggestion or my little tantrum/pep talk, but suddenly, 90 percent of my class was saying the affirmations! The energy in the room immediately shifted; you could feel this powerful, positive energy vibrating all around us. By the end of class, many people were surprised by their emotional state. Many of them were crying. "What happened?" they wanted to know. Why this burst of emotion, this release of tension? It's simple: relief. If you are someone who is really hard on yourself, constantly comparing yourself to others and never feeling good enough, then when you do something different (like this workout), you feel relief from the negativity and the harsh words. It's an incredible feeling, a high.

When you learn to exercise and keep your mind in a positive state, encouraging yourself instead of discouraging yourself, you can feel the alignment happening between what you want, what you are thinking, and what you are doing. During a workout, you usually feel your heart pounding, your breath deepening, your muscles burning. But when your mind is on the goal and you are deliberately calling up your courage, your strength, your willpower, your faith, and your self-respect, you are not feeling any of the strain or pain. You are not praying for the workout to be over every minute you are doing it. You are not watching a clock or groaning, moaning, or complaining. You will find you can go longer and harder, and the workout no longer feels like work. It's an empowering choice, not a chore.

You, too, may feel skeptical, unwilling, and downright ridiculous saying these affirmations, especially if you have been having a very different conversation with yourself. You'll get over it. Say the affirmation silently if you have to at first; then build to a whisper, a statement, a shout. Eventually all your hesitation will melt away—especially when you see the results. But understand this: When I tell you to speak out loud, it's not just mouthing the words. When people use affirmations without emotion or motion, they have very little effect. You are embody-ing these words: Be them, emotionalize them, act upon them. Feel the words fueling you. It's like being supercharged. Find your warrior voice. Be the change you seek! Your time has come.

Excuses, Excuses

After teaching hundreds of classes over fifteen years, I have heard them all. Sometimes it's utterly shocking how people find a way to "negative-ize" even a positive workout. They feel good when they leave the class; they feel different. Uh-oh . . . here comes that fear and self-doubt creeping up again. I hear:

"If I can't work out for an hour, what's the point?"
"If I am going to lose only a pound a week, why should I even try?"
"I'll never be able to stick to this."

All these statements, my friend, are cop-outs. Remember, change is the accumulation of steps you take in one direction or another. You will not achieve success in one big, explosive moment. It will come over time, with consistent action over time.

Instead, try saying:

"What I can do is enough because it is all I can do and it is enough."

"I will be thrilled to lose a pound a week instead of gaining a pound a week."

"I am willing to do this now more than ever before."

Let's play a little game of "Patricia Says." The first statements are those of the whiner; see how I substitute them with a more positive statement—the words of the warrior. Try it yourself.

"I don't have time."
Patricia says: **"I can always find the time."**

"My family won't support me."
Patricia says: **"I will be an inspiration to my family, and I'll influence their health positively."**

"It's my vacation/birthday/his birthday/her birthday."
Patricia says: **"If I am prepared, then I won't be tempted."**

"I am traveling all the time; it's impossible to keep it up."
Patricia says: **"I can pack foods that are good for me to travel with."**

I used to use the traveling excuse a lot. I traveled once a month, often out of the country. I felt that what I ate at the airport, on the plane, or in another country didn't count! Well, it counted—and the scale counted all the pounds I was putting on by ditching my desire on the road. I remember going to teach at a convention in Siberia, and, having just made a new promise to myself to eat well, I decided to pack a bag of things I could eat, wanted to eat, and would be willing to eat. I felt in control; I felt proud of myself. I had made a different choice, and no longer could I use the excuse "I travel too much." I was empowered! It was not easy taking the extra time to pack (or taking the extra luggage!), but since then, I have seen myself as able to handle difficult situations differently. I also proved to myself that I really *did* care. It felt great.

Building New Muscle

Start by making a list of actions that you would feel proud of yourself for doing. Make the list as long as you can. Write things down that are absolutely easy for you to do that you can do now, as well as things you would like to get yourself to do *eventually* but are not ready to do just yet.

Make a list of daily as well as weekly actions that will support you in fulfilling your goal. Now you can see and appreciate every little step you take in the right direction. You can begin to view yourself differently. You are building your action-taking muscle. This list should represent things that you will *absolutely* commit to. It also gives you the chance to notice if you are taking action with integrity and if you are activating the whiner or the warrior voice.

Here is an example of an action list:

WHAT CAN I DO *DAILY* TO SUPPORT MY GOAL OF LOSING 5 POUNDS THIS MONTH?

❋ Drink eight glasses of water.
❋ Eat two pieces of fruit.
❋ Eat two cups of salad.
❋ Eat three meals.
❋ No skipping breakfast.
❋ No eating after 6 p.m.
❋ Journal for five minutes in the morning.
❋ Cut out white-flour carbs.
❋ Post my success sheet in a place that will remind me daily of my goals.
❋ Check off my list daily.
❋ Write down five reasons why I am proud of myself each day.

WHAT CAN I DO *WEEKLY* TO SUPPORT MY GOAL OF LOSING 5 POUNDS THIS MONTH?

❋ Do a cardio workout three times a week for a minimum of 30 minutes, no matter what.

❋ Do my favorite yoga DVD at home at least once.

❋ Walk instead of taking a bus/cab/car at least once a week.

❋ Take the stairs instead of the elevator at least once a week.

❋ Compliment myself every time I achieve a goal.

❋ Say this affirmation at least once a week, out loud:

> *Inspired action is the key to my success*
> *And positive thoughts fuel my action best!*
> *I have courage, confidence, love, and compassion,*
> *I am worth it today; I am taking action.*

FUEL YOUR SUCCESS

I will act now.
I am strong now.
I am confident now.
All negative thoughts
Stop right now!

Do each move for at least one minute before going on to the next move, so you can get the maximum benefit.

You will feel this exercise in your upper body, but also in your waist. If you exaggerate the twisting action of this move, your abs will applaud you and you will feel the heat in your body rising. This is a very good sign. Don't stop until you feel you can no longer speak or no longer hold your arms up. Get your heart pumping and the sweat pouring! Don't give up too soon, or you will miss the benefit! When you get yourself to the point of fatigue, you are telling your body you want more strength. In order to get more strength, you have to use what you have. Feel it in your core. This is an awesome exercise for your arms, your core, and your mental strength. Go for it. Don't stop until you have to. Use the strength you have now; it's enough.

SAY, "I WILL ACT NOW."

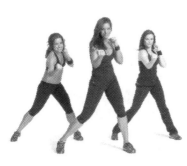

Stand in the On-Guard position: legs hip width apart, elbows bent and close to your body, fists at either side of your chin. Keeping your elbows bent, punch your right fist up toward the center of your body, allowing your torso to rotate slightly to the left. Return to the On-Guard position.

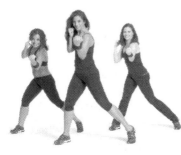

Repeat on the other side. Punch your left fist toward the center of your body, allowing your torso to rotate to the right. Remember to return to the On-Guard position after each punch.

STRONG

SAY, "I AM STRONG NOW."

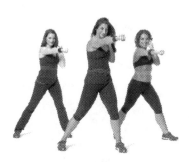

Stand in the On-Guard position. Punch your right fist across your body, your palm facing down, allowing your torso to rotate slightly. Return to the On-Guard position.

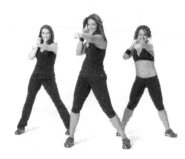

Repeat on the other side. Remember to keep your elbows pointing toward the floor and your palms facing down. Return to the On-Guard position after each punch.

CONFIDENT

SAY, "I AM CONFIDENT NOW."

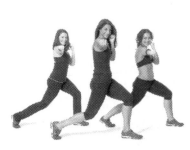

Stand in the On-Guard position. Pivot to your left, bending your knees in a lunge position (keep your left foot flat on the floor and allow your right heel to come off), and punch your right fist 2 times in a double pump toward center.

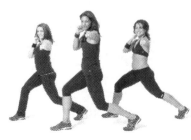

In one motion, pivot to the right and repeat on the other side, punching your left fist 2 times in a double pump toward center. Fully extend each arm in the double punch, and remember to return your arms to the On-Guard position after each double punch.

SELF-CONTROL

SAY, "ALL NEGATIVE THOUGHTS"

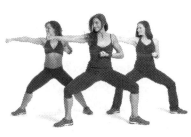

Stand in a straight-leg Warrior stance. With bent elbows, place your right forearm over your left forearm in front of your body. In one motion, bend your knees in the Warrior stance and open your arms, extending your right arm directly to your right side as the left fist slides back by your left shoulder, as if you are shooting a bow and arrow.

When you master yourself, you will master your life. When you find yourself able to say, "That's it! No more negativity!" you will feel empowered and free. Imagine in this exercise hugging yourself first, and then extending one arm out. Alternate which hand is on top during the hug. The arm on top is the one that will extend. The core is key in this exercise. Hold your abs in, and when you extend your arms out to the side, make sure the arms stop in line with your body, not behind your body. The more you bend your knees, the more challenging it is. Do your best to contract the muscles of your biceps and triceps instead of locking your elbows. If you make a strong fist, it will help you engage the muscles in your arms. Feel the warrior spirit coming out of you! Make sure you are doing what you are saying. If you are feeling better, you are thinking better thoughts. Well done!

SELF-CONTROL

SAY, "STOP RIGHT NOW!"

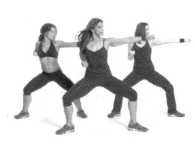

Return to the straight-leg Warrior stance and place your left forearm arm over your right forearm in front of your body. Again, in one motion, bend your knees the in Warrior stance and open your arms, extending your left arm directly to your left side as the right fist slides back by your left shoulder, as if shooting a strong and powerful arrow.

Remember to keep the palm of your fist facing down to the floor as the arm extends, and don't let it overextend behind you.

SERIES BREAKDOWN

After you have done each exercise for at least one minute, it's time to break down the series and run it through.

Say, "I will act now, I am strong now."

"I will act now"—INSPIRED. Alternate punching your arms up toward your chin for 8 counts.

- "I" (punch right and left for 2 counts)
- "will" (punch right and left for 2 counts)
- "act" (punch right and left for 2 counts)
- "now" (punch right and left for 2 counts)

"I am strong now"—STRENGTH. Punch in front of you for 8 counts.

- "I" (punch right and left for 2 counts)
- "am" (punch right and left for 2 counts)
- "strong" (punch right and left for 2 counts)
- "now" (punch right and left for 2 counts)

Run through the entire phrase for one to two minutes:

- "I will act now"—COMMITMENT (8 counts)
- "I am strong now"—STRENGTH (8 counts)

Say, "I am confident now. All negative thoughts stop right now."

"I am confident now"—CONFIDENCE. Double punches right and left for 8 counts.

- "I" (double punch right for 2 counts)
- "am" (double punch left for 2 counts)
- "confident" (double punch right for 2 counts)
- "now" (double punch left for 2 counts)

"All negative thoughts stop right now"—SELF-CONTROL.

Alternate shooting your arms like an arrow right and left for 8 counts.

- "All negative" (shoot arm to the right for 2 counts)
- "thoughts" (shoot arm to the left for 2 counts)
- "stop" (shoot arm to the right for 2 counts)
- "right now" (shoot arm to the right for 2 counts)

Run through just these two moves for one to two minutes:

- "I am confident now"—CONFIDENCE (8 counts)
- "All negative thoughts stop right now"— SELF-CONTROL (8 counts)

Run through the whole series from the top:

- "I will act now"—COMMITMENT (8 counts)
- "I am strong now"—STRENGTH (8 counts)
- "I am confident now"—CONFIDENCE (8 counts)

"All negative thoughts stop right now"—SELF-CONTROL (8 counts)

CHAPTER CHECKLIST
i will . . .

* Practice being who I want to be. I will act, walk, talk, eat, live as if I have already succeeded.

* Remember a time in my life when I was successful and how good it felt to follow through on my commitment to myself.

* Catch my excuses! Every time I make an excuse, I will stop and realize that I am deflating my power.

DISCIPLINE IS NOT A PUNISHMENT— IT'S A REWARD

All of the suggestions I have given you so far are useful—*if* you can get yourself to do them. Now we come to one of the most important parts of the IntenSati program—the glue, so to speak, that holds it all together: discipline.

I know, I know . . . the word sends shivers down your spine. It sounds so rigid, dictating, tough. Like an army drill sergeant or your mean third-grade math teacher. No one wants to be told what to do; no one likes to be bossed around. No one likes to feel tied, constrained, or limited. The word brings up great resistance and fear in many people—it is something to rebel against or run away from.

But I am here to tell you the opposite is true. Discipline is freedom. It is you getting yourself to do what you really want to do.

You are your own boss. *You* set the rules and make sure you follow through on them. Discipline empowers you to be the master rather than the slave. Discipline allows you to see the bigger picture, even when something yummy is looming in front of you. Here's an example: Every day, you head out of your office at three o'clock for a coffee break. You buy yourself a large, frosty iced coffee drink—you know the kind I mean: topped with whipped cream and caramel syrup! "Hey," you reason, "it's not really food if I can drink it. And I really *need* it to get through the rest of my day."

So here is my question to you: Do you *really* need it? Is your life, your job, your mental and physical and emotional wellness dependent on that huge 300-calorie coffee? "Well," you respond, "I'm addicted to it. I can't give it up." Oh, really? You can't? Is there someone grabbing your hand and forcing that straw to your lips? What you are lacking here, my friend, is the discipline to stick to your goals. Remember to think of what you are gaining, instead of what you are giving up. Hold fast to the goal, the dream, the desire to feel better, to have more energy, to feel lighter, healthier, more self-confident, instead of giving in to five minutes of pleasure. Holding on to this vision—not just resisting the treat—is discipline at its most empowering. You're looking at the short term—the here and now: that sugary drink is calling, and you want immediate gratification. Don't let yourself down; stop and think for a moment from your heart.

What if I told you that giving up that afternoon coffee for just one month would save you almost 6,000 calories? And that—even without any exercise—those saved calories would translate into losing 2 to 3 pounds? And that if you kept it up for a year, you could lose as much as 36 pounds? Would that change your mind?

So what will you do tomorrow at three o'clock when you feel slouchy and tired and your craving is kicking into high gear? How are you going to stop yourself from getting up and having your coffee drink? Simple: Have a Plan B. Something that you can do (or eat or drink) that will make you feel better without derailing your intentions. To deprive yourself entirely would be cruel and unusual punishment (and will eventually backfire). Instead, think of a better way, a smarter way, to satisfy your craving. Think of a way to honor your intentions and make the right choice.

You could:

* Remind yourself that being able to do what you said you would do is the goal.
* Drink two large glasses of water. This will perk you up if you are dehydrated.
* Remind yourself not to let yourself down—this is for you. Say to yourself, "This is a test of my will, and I will pass!"
* Tell yourself this is not a punishment, but a reward. Tell yourself, "Discipline is my reward!"
* Avoid temptation: Don't go into the coffee place. Go for a quick walk around the block and breathe some fresh air.
* Review your vision board.
* Have a small square of dark organic chocolate.
* Have a bottle or two of flavored water.
* Have some fresh fruit.
* Call or e-mail someone to catch up.
* Close your eyes and imagine yourself succeeding.

What Is Self-Discipline?

First, I will tell you what discipline is *not*. It is not a punishment for being overweight and letting yourself get out of shape. It is not depriving yourself or beating yourself up. It is not sucking all the joy out of your life. Discipline is not saying no for the sake of torturing yourself. It is not about starving, sulking, or stewing.

Discipline is present inside all of us. As we feed our self-discipline, we grow stronger, braver, more awake and aware of the possibility of a new way of life. It takes time, patience, and love to develop.

* ❋ Self-discipline means holding fast to your vision of health and happiness and acting, moment by moment, with integrity in order to achieve that vision.
* ❋ Self-discipline empowers you to surrender negative thoughts for positive ones.
* ❋ Self-discipline motivates you to get off the couch and go to the gym, even when you don't feel like it.
* ❋ Self-discipline allows you to choose fresh food over easier fast food.
* ❋ Self-discipline means honoring yourself enough to know that you deserve to feel and live better.
* ❋ Self-discipline means engaging honestly and deeply with any fears, failures, and old habits currently standing in your way.
* ❋ Self-discipline grants you the power to keep your word in the face of any challenge.
* ❋ Self-discipline is freedom, abundance, joy, and happiness—not punishment, restraint, and suffering.

When you hold your attention unconditionally on your vision of what you want, you loosen your inner hold on the old ways of immediate gratification: the junk food or the TV instead of the workout. It may be really hard for you to hold fast to that dream when a craving comes on or you really *do* feel tired. But it is in those very challenging moments, the ones where you are going back and forth with yourself about what to do, whether to keep to your action plan or give it up, that you must stop and realize you are fighting for something you don't want anymore: It is just an old habit. If you choose to take the high road, that feeling of empowerment will fuel your entire life.

Arguing with Ourselves

Have you ever seen a mother and child arguing? The child screams, "I want it!" and the mother responds, "Not now." This goes back and forth, three, four, even five times and then . . . the mother gives in, because the child's tantrum gets too big to handle. She's exhausted. She can't stand to hear the whining anymore. We play this tug-of-war within ourselves as well. When we don't have a relationship to our commitments and promises, we whine and complain, just like that bratty kid—and then we just give in and give up. If you have had this conversation with yourself before and "lost" many times, it will determine how strong you are the next time at following through.

We train ourselves, just as we train our children. If the child knows that "no" really means "if I throw a big enough tantrum it will be yes," then the child learns to get what he wants by whining. But if the mother holds firm, and the child knows that "no" means "no," the tantrums magically stop. The child learns to shift his or her attention to something else. When you stop giving your attention to the whining voices, they disappear. The result is the exhilarating emergence of personal power. The warrior is now in charge!

You also have the amazing ability to turn a "no!" into a "yes!" Have you ever told yourself, "Today I will not have any bread!" What happens? You spend the whole day obsessing over it; you have bread on the brain! Every window you look into, every storefront you pass, seems to be selling you *exactly* what you have sworn off. Your eyes will keep seeing and smelling and mentally tasting the warm bagel, the perfect sandwich, the pizza, the basket of rolls on the dinner table. Why? Because when you say "no" to something, you register it on your radar. It is taking up your attention. When I was taking a 12-step program for "food addicts," we weren't even allowed to mention the "forbidden" foods to one another. The very mention of one of these "nos" could lead us to fantasize about it—and eat it. Imagine, simply saying a word can have the power to make that craving come to life!

Well, how about we use this powerful principle to our advantage? If it works so well when we say "no!" to something, then how about if you say "yes!" to something else instead? Make yourself a list, the longer the better, of all the healthy choices you can eat: the sweet, juicy fruits and healthy, crunchy salads. All the foods you *can* eat. Now imagine yourself enjoying each food: smell it, taste it, imagine it, envision it, live it. The longer your list, the more the choices will feel inspiring instead of deflating.

Sometimes you make a promise to yourself and you just can't keep it. It happens. You were going to go work out and your babysitter didn't show. Or you got called in to work or your trainer canceled or you're too darn tired. What do you do now? You do the best you can. You remember what you want, and you decide to work out at home, or go after work, or you make sure you work out tomorrow, which was supposed to be your day off.

The promises you make to yourself are your ticket to a new life. They are little exercises of self-love, personal power, and commitment. You know when you are lying to yourself. You can feel it in your gut: It feels like guilt, worry, fear, or anger. Fulfill your promise

> ### Words to live by
>
> *What you have done is unimportant compared to what you are about to do.*
>
> *How you have erred is insignificant compared to how you are about to create.*

another way or just simply do the best you can do with the situation you have. Think like a warrior! Where there is a will, there is a way. Tell yourself, "I will find a way," instead of just giving up. When you succeed in these moments, you feel proud, and that confidence will fuel your whole life.

Practicing Your Power

Strengthening your discipline is like learning a new language or a new skill. At first it's awkward, strange, and even uncomfortable. Picture a child learning to ride a bike for the first time: she wobbles, she stops and starts, she falls. Do you just shout at her, "Oh well, I guess you're just not cut out to ride a bike." Of course not! You cheer her on until she finds her courage and her balance.

It's the same with self-discipline. You have to encourage yourself instead of discourage yourself and know that self-discipline is a valuable characteristic, one worth developing. It will benefit your entire life, not just this one area.

In the same way that you applaud a child for getting back up on a bike and continuing to try, applaud yourself for fumbling through your developing self-discipline. Every time you succeed at keeping a commitment to yourself, give yourself a standing ovation instead of condemning yourself for falling down. Pat yourself on the back when you make changes. Celebrate and pay attention to the feelings of empowerment small changes provide, and notice how different you feel when you make choices that are in alignment with what you really want.

Each act of self-discipline, no matter how small, is like building a fortress, brick by brick. You say no to the vending machine today. It's hard; you want that candy bar *bad*. But you do it because you said you would. The next day, passing that vending machine, you glance at that gooey chocolaty treat and it's a little easier to walk on by. The next day, you barely even see the candy machine, and it gets easier and easier as your self-discipline grows.

To build your muscle of self-discipline, you're going to start by making yourself a little "promises journal" to practice making promises to yourself and keeping them.

1. Keep your vision clear in your mind and remember why you want to achieve this vision. Start each day looking at your vision board and looking forward to your inspiring future.

2. Remind yourself you are here to thrive, not just survive.

3. Write down, "I love myself enough to improve my attitude."

4. In the morning, write down "I will have _____ for lunch today." No matter what, *have it*—even if you are craving something else.

5. Pick one thing to add to your diet: more fruit, water, vegetables, and other healthy things. Define how much you will add, and no matter what, do your best to follow through.

6. Choose a food you want to eliminate from your diet for one day, one week, one month. Write it down. No matter what, do your best to succeed.

7. Pick an action you will add to your life, such as journaling, writing down everything you eat, meditating, planning your day. Also, choose how often or

how long you will do it. No matter what, do your best to succeed.

8. Pick an exercise you will add to your life. Be specific about what it is, how long you will do it, how many times you will do it, and how often. No matter what, do your best to succeed.

9. Stop yourself from whining and throwing tantrums about the process. Tell people you know will support you and your goal. Ask them to remind you when they hear you whining about "having to" go work out or "having to" lose weight or "having to" eat better. Remember, you don't "have to" do anything. This is your choice. This is your power.

10. If you find you are just not able to fulfill a promise (it was too much for you), before you break it, sit down and rewrite it. For example, if you promised not to eat the candy bar at three o'clock today and you couldn't resist, then write, "I will have this now, and I will run 20 minutes this evening." Or "I will have this now but then I won't have the glass of wine at dinner I was going to have." Keep the renegotiated promise.

11. Finally, forgive yourself. When you make a choice that goes against your original promise, let yourself off the hook. Say it and write it: "I forgive me." And get up and try again!

MIND/BODY EXERCISE:
THE FREEDOM OF DISCIPLINE

I am that.
I am free.
I discipline
My attention
To harness the power
Of concentration.

The words you say after the words "I am . . ." are very powerful. You are declaring who you are, who you have been, or who you choose to be. Pay attention. Go as low as you can go, and feel your hamstrings and buttocks working. When you feel your muscles burning and you really want to stop, do one more! Don't slouch; keep a powerful, positive posture at all times. Practice each move one at a time until you feel comfortable with the moves and the vocabulary. Then do Part 2; you are about to experience the lower-body part of the practice. This part of the workout will shape your lower body beautifully. It will help you develop incredible balance and at the same time work your core muscles. Challenge yourself!

GRATITUDE

SAY, "I AM"

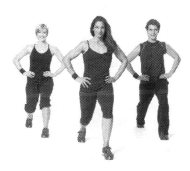

Step your right foot behind you to a rear lunge, keeping your left foot flat on the floor and your right heel raised. Tuck your pelvis under and your abs in, and place your hands on your hips.

INFINITE POTENTIAL

SAY, "THAT."

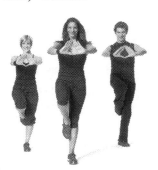

Push up to a single-leg balance, bending your right knee up to hip level. Place your hands in the triangle mudra (your thumbs and index fingers touch) in front of your heart.

The triangle shape made by your hands represents that you are infinite potential. When your thoughts, actions, and attitude are in positive alignment, anything is possible. Keep your standing leg straight and imagine pushing the floor away so you can rise up.

GRATITUDE

SAY, "I AM"

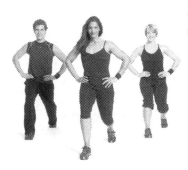

Return to a rear lunge on the same side.

PEACE

SAY, "FREE."

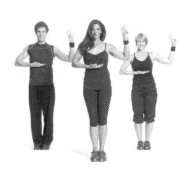

Come up and stand with your feet together. With your upper arm parallel to the floor, bend your elbow and make a "peace" sign with your right hand. Cup your left hand just below your heart and stand tall.

DISCIPLINE

SAY, "I"

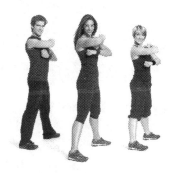

Step to the right diagonal, your arms in a chamber position (right forearm over left forearm) in front of your body.

SAY, "DISCIPLINE"

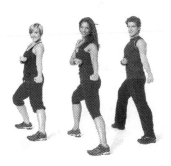

Bend your right knee and turn out your right foot, keeping your knee over the ankle and both feet flat on the floor. Simultaneously extend and rotate your left arm down and away from the body. Your right fist slides back toward the left shoulder, opening the chest.

When you are able to discipline your mind, you will harness your most powerful asset: your creative energy. Imagine you are protecting your body from something coming at you as you lean back and get out of the way. Feel the warrior spirit in you. Do as many as exercises you can. How do you know when to stop? When your legs are burning! Handling a challenging situation takes discipline and strength. You are building both. Do your best.

ATTENTION

SAY, "MY ATTENTION"

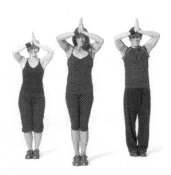

Step your feet together. With your palms touching (Prayer position), place the heels of your hands on the center of your forehead, at the third eye.

With this move, you are touching your "third eye," the eye of your imagination. It is your creative eye, because what you think about, you bring about. Careful not to cover your eyes with your hands! Keep your gaze straight ahead. If you are having a hard time balancing, focus on one thing in front of you.

POWER

SAY, "TO HARNESS THE POWER"

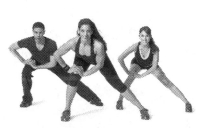

From a standing position, powerfully step to the right into a deep lunge with your right leg, keeping your back straight and allowing the buttocks to reach back. Your feet are parallel and flat on the floor. Reach your left arm to the floor and place your right arm on your right thigh for support. Look straight ahead.

To modify the pose, take a moderate lunge and place both hands on your thigh.

CONCENTRATION

SAY, "OF CONCENTRATION."

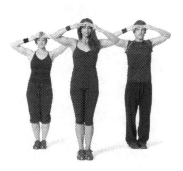

From the lunge, push off and return and bring your feet together. Place the first three fingers of both hands on your forehead.

SERIES BREAKDOWN

Say, "I am that" (GRATITUDE / INFINITE POTENTIAL)
- "I am"—GRATITUDE. Rear lunge with hands on hips.
- "that"—INFINITE POTENTIAL. Single-leg balance, hands in triangle position.

Combine the two moves on the right side only for one minute, then on the left side only for one minute, then alternate right and left for one minute.

Say, "I am free" (GRATITUDE / PEACE)
- "I am"—GRATITUDE. Rear lunge with hands on hips.
- "free"—PEACE. Single-leg balance, hand makes a peace sign.

Combine the two moves on the right side only for one minute, then on the left side only for one minute, then alternate right and left for one minute.

Now run through the series from the top. "I am that, I am free"
- "I am that"—GRATITUDE / INFINITE POTENTIAL
- "I am free"—GRATITUDE / PEACE

First run through 8 times on the right side, then 8 times on the left, then alternate 8 times right and left.

Say, "I discipline my attention" (DISCIPLINE / ATTENTION)
- "I discipline"—DISCIPLINE. Side block with the arm.
- "my attention"—ATTENTION. Hands are in the Prayer position, touching the forehead.

Combine the two moves on the right side only for one minute, then on the left side only for one minute, then alternate right and left for one minute.

Say, "To harness my power of concentration" (POWER / CON-CENTRATION)

- "To harness my power"—POWER. Step to a deep side lunge.
- "of concentration"—CONCENTRATION. Standing in a single-leg balance, press three fingers of each hand on your forehead.

Combine these two moves on the right side only for one minute, then on the left side only for one minute, then alternate right and left for one minute.

Now say, "I discipline my attention to harness the power of concentration."

- "I discipline my attention"—DISCIPLINE / ATTENTION
- "to harness my power of concentration"—POWER / CONCENTRATION

First run through 8 times on the right side, then 8 times on the left, then alternate 8 times right and left.

Now run through the entire series from the top. First run through the series 8 times on the right side, then 8 times on the left, then alternate 8 times right and left.

- "I am that"—GRATITUDE / INFINITE POTENTIAL
- "I am free"—GRATITUDE / PEACE
- "I discipline my attention"—DISCIPLINE / ATTENTION
- "to harness my power of concentration"—POWER / CONCENTRATION

CHAPTER CHECKLIST

i Will...

❋ Remind myself that self-discipline is a reward—not a punishment.

❋ Make a long list of all the healthy things I can eat, instead of dwelling on the bad foods I should give up.

❋ Forgive myself if I go against my promise. Vow to do better next time.

principle six

LOVE IS THE ENGINE
OF SUCCESS

I want you to be totally honest with yourself. When was the last time you walked down the street, caught a glimpse of your reflection in a store window, and thought, "Wow, I look great!"? When did you last look forward to shopping for a new bathing suit—or even stepping out of a dressing room to share the mirror with other people? How long has it been since you took a spot in the front row of your workout or yoga class and didn't feel self-conscious? If you're scratching your head, struggling to recall a moment when you didn't *despise* yourself, I have the answer: Love is all you need. Most of the time, we dismiss love as a warm and fuzzy emotion—the stuff that Hallmark cards and mushy songs on the radio are made of. But love has enormous power. If you can learn to stop loathing yourself and start loving yourself, you will unlock the secret to having everything you desire—and then some.

Think of how it feels when you're in love with someone, how the powerful, positive emotions envelop you and make you feel as if you're floating on air. It's illuminating, euphoric, indisputably the best feeling in the world. What if you could look at yourself through those eyes? What if the next time you gazed in the mirror you saw someone you adored and appreciated? "Impossible!" you say, "I have ten, twenty, thirty pounds I need to lose—and what about that cellulite?" Change your point of view to a more loving one! If you are willing to see yourself as a human being with challenges, fears, successes, and failures, instead of defining yourself by how much you weigh this day, this week, or this month, your ability to love will expand. And when you are feeling that giddiness about life, about your present moment and your future, you will have the fuel to face the changes—and the power to take action.

My (self) Love Story

I wasn't always in love with love. I once read a self-help book that recommended you look in the mirror and declare "I love you." Well, I mulled it over—and then I totally rejected the idea. I thought it was absolutely ridiculous. What difference would telling myself "I love you" make? Besides, of course I loved myself! Everyone loves themselves . . . don't they? What really bugged me—and continued to for days—was that I had such a cynical reaction to this seemingly innocuous advice. I rolled my eyes and scoffed at the absurdity of it. It even made me mad. Why? Because I knew, deep down, that I had fallen out of love with myself.

The problem became crystal clear to me on a photo shoot shortly afterward. I was questioning whether I had lost enough weight to be photographed in exercise clothes (spandex is not very forgiving). As the day progressed, my bad mood kept inflating like a balloon. My joy was fading fast, and the closer I got to the hour of the shoot, the more I doubted myself. "Okay, Patricia," I tried to reason, "why are you beating yourself up? Whose approval are you looking for here?" I had been written up in at least fifty magazines; I had won numerous fitness awards; I had done more than fifteen workout videos. On a personal level, I was in love and had a perfect partner and was making a great living. I had already achieved many of the things I had been working toward, so when was it going to be enough? Was I *really* going to let all I had and all I had accomplished be meaningless?

Who was it who had to crown me "good enough"? I already had the job. What weight did I have to be? Was it worth sacrificing my joy for 10 pounds? I asked myself point-blank, "What will be enough to convince you?" If I am on *Oprah,* does that mean I am good enough? If my classes get more packed, if I do another video, am I good enough? If I get the cover of a magazine? When does this end? I realized it was a battle that was truly *never* going to end unless I was willing to approve of myself and not seek everyone else's blessing.

The shoot was not my best work. I was extremely self-conscious, and it was so unlike me. Usually, I love being in front of the camera. But this time, I didn't shine. I tried to crowd out my negative self and get back to the place I knew felt good and right, but that day I couldn't do it. I let the criticizing voice deplete my energy. The results were less than impressive: my smile was forced; my poses were uninspiring. I was unhappy, and it showed. I kept comparing myself to everyone else, and it was a very painful experience. When I left, I promised myself that I would deal with whatever was making me so miserable. If I wanted to do what I loved (teaching exercise), if I wanted to find that self-confident place again, I had to figure out what the problem was.

I didn't have to look very far to see what was knocking my self-confidence for a loop: I had gained weight, and, worse, I had ignored it. I had not shown up at this shoot at my best, and I tortured myself every minute because of it. I had so many good excuses for *why* I had gained the weight: I had an injury, and I couldn't work out; I had been traveling, which made it hard to eat well; it was a last-minute job and I didn't have time to prepare . . . it went on and on and on. All perfectly good excuses—great ones, in fact. But that's all they were—excuses. The only thing that mattered now was that I didn't love who I was. I had to choose to get back in the game, find a better plan, and do what I really wanted to do, which was feel my best again.

So I went back to training, mentally and physically. I got real about the fact that I was not okay at this weight and realized that agonizing over these 10 extra pounds was costing me my happiness. I shifted my attention off waiting to receive love and took the responsibility of giving it to myself. It felt so much better—as if a huge cloud had lifted. I changed my goal from "I want to be thin" to "I want to feel good and to love who I am." Although it wasn't an overnight success (the 10 pounds didn't drop off immediately), I felt instant relief. I realized how just making the decision to get myself back on track was a loving choice. I could see myself with renewed appreciation and admiration—even with those extra pounds—because I was acting out of love and integrity. And yes, I did lose the weight, but what I gained was an incredible feeling of empowerment.

Nobody's Perfect

Everyone is unique, and we all have certain body parts that we struggle with. We're human; we're not perfect. Not everyone is willing to do what it takes to have washboard abs or ripped biceps or even cellulite-free thighs. When we embrace ourselves 100 percent, we stop trying to hide our "flaws" and fit into an idea of what we think others will love or accept. But until we accept who we are and where we are in our own life, we will not have access to the energy of love within us that will help us to see ourselves differently. Unless you are willing to love, accept, and forgive yourself, you will forever look outside yourself for approval or acceptance from others. Think about it: You can't "hate yourself" thin or complain away your pain. It takes action to reach both those objectives. Love is that action. It is the fuel that ignites your courage, helps you face your fear, and opens your eyes to new possibilities. You cannot take loving action from a place of hate, shame, guilt, or disappointment.

Ask yourself this: "What do I really care about? What is really important to me?" If the answer is "my body, my health, my willpower and discipline," then the loving gesture is to face it, work on it, and resolve it, so it is no longer something you can use against yourself. Instead of whining about what you *can't* achieve, define what you really care about achieving—then go for it! Fuel your success with love, and love yourself enough to improve your lifestyle, your mood, and your attitude.

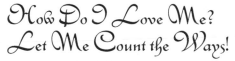

How Do I Love Me? Let Me Count the Ways!

Love starts in the mirror and grows from there. It is a process that takes nurturing. It won't happen overnight. Once you are able to look at yourself with love and appreciation, you need to live each day embodying that love. The way you take care of yourself—how you eat, if you exercise, how you speak, what you choose to do as a career or a form of self-expression—speaks volumes, not only to others but to your own self. Love is not always taking the path of least resistance or the easy way out. It is about checking in with yourself and finding out what is important to you, then living up to your values. It has nothing to do with what anyone else thinks of you and everything to do with what *you* think about you. Loving yourself is not ignoring a problem or quelling it with food, drink, sleep, or other things. Loving yourself is taking action to help youself reach your fullest potential. You will always find your best self when you choose to love. But

OPEN YOUR HEART

Though at first I scoffed at this exercise, I now ask my students to face the mirror and declare their love for themselves. The first time they do it, you can feel the squirming in the room. Some people look down at their feet; others snicker or roll their eyes; one or two have actually walked out! There are also a few who cry, proving how deeply moving and powerful this exercise can be. It is a softening of the heart that allows those tears to flow and helps you realize how far from feeling love you have been. When you feel this amazing moment, you will wonder how you let yourself get so far away from it in the first place.

This exercise is about opening your heart and connecting to the feeling of love. Take a few moments to stop and be with yourself and your breath. The more you do it, the easier it gets. At first, it may be just a whisper, but eventually you will be able to celebrate yourself and sing your praises from the rooftops! Are you ready?

Face the mirror. Look into your eyes. Look into your heart. Say silently to yourself:

"I love and accept myself exactly as I am."

How does it feel to think these words? Now say them aloud. How does it feel to speak them?

When you are declaring that you love and accept yourself and you *don't,* something feels very "off." You feel awkward, cynical, disconnected. This is a great warning sign, a time to stop and ask yourself:

❋ Why is this so hard?
❋ Why do I have such a negative reaction to this?
❋ Why does this feel corny or fake, rather than true?
❋ What is it that I am not happy with?
❋ Am I willing to change what I cannot accept and accept what I cannot change?

If looking in the mirror is challenging for you, try this: Find a friend you can work with. Stand face-to-face and just look each other in the eyes without saying anything. Mentally say to each other, "I love you." Don't actually utter the words; just feel what happens. You may start to laugh and giggle, but that is just your discomfort and a way to avoid feeling vulnerable. But if you stay with it a little longer, giving your attention to the other person and feeling how he or she is breathing, just being there in the silence together . . . something beautiful will happen. You will see the humanity of the other person. It is an indescribable feeling, and it's different every time you do it, depending on the partner you choose. Because it takes courage to sit there quietly, it will help you experience that beautiful connection to love that sometimes is hard to feel on your own. And when you feel it, you will definitely know! There is a sense of relief, of freedom, of present-moment awareness. Time stops, and for a moment the mind chattering stops; all you feel is joy and appreciation. Bask in the glow!

you must love yourself enough to improve your actions and attitude, and to tell the truth.

You're going to create your own "Love Myself" to-do list:

* Pay attention to yourself. Start noticing how often you are grumpy, cranky, uninspired, or tired. Care enough about yourself that you are not willing to live in this unhappy state. Check in with yourself and get curious about *why* you are not happy, why you are feeling less than your best. Don't ignore it; it's a sign that you need/want some attention.

* Make a list of all the things that are bothering you. Write down all your complaints, every single one of them that you can think of. Then cross the ones off

your list that can't do anything about (your age, your height, your parents, and so on), and circle the ones you will take action on one day but not now. Finally, put a date next to the ones you will deal with; give yourself realistic deadlines. Don't worry about the how; just focus for now on the commitment to take care of them. The how will reveal itself.

❋ Take inspired action. Figure out what you can do now to move you in the direction you want to go and *do it*! You will feel tremendous relief the moment you start taking loving action.

❋ Remember, you are the only one who is holding love back from you, and you can give it back to yourself at any time. Journal, exercise, make a healthy meal, clean out all the junk food from your fridge. A single positive action can inspire!

❋ Be courageous! Do the things that you haven't done because you are afraid of disappointment or rejection. Go on a date or a job interview. Buy yourself a sexy little black dress and choose to feel sexy in it.

❋ If you need some support (as most of us do), hire a life coach to help you gain the strength to get to your truth. (I recommend The Handel Group: coach@ handelgroup.com.) A life coach is someone who helps you figure out the best way for you to achieve the things you are having a hard time figuring out on your own. Lauren, the founder of the Handel method, worked with me on starting my business, falling in love, dealing with my personal integrity, and finding the courage to speak and live my truth. The Handel Group also coached my sister to a 150-pound weight loss!

* Make a list of all your dreams, the small ones and the big ones, and ask yourself if you are using your weight as an excuse not to go for them. If you are, deal with your weight so you can live your dream.

* Write yourself a letter of apology and forgiveness: "I am sorry for not taking better care of you. Please forgive me for not treating you with respect and compassion . . ." End it with loving promises to improve.

MIND/BODY EXERCISE: LOVE IS ALL YOU NEED

All I need
Is within me now
For my life
All others
And myself.
I accept and I love myself
Exactly as I am

EMBRACE

SAY, "ALL I NEED"

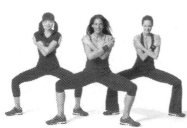

Step to the right into Warrior legs and give yourself a big hug.

Hug yourself and really feel it. You are reminding yourself that you have everything you need. Really feel the sweetness of this move. Your legs will burn with this exercise if you do it long enough. Go through and practice each move one at a time until you know the moves and the vocabulary.

POSITIVE EXPECTATION

SAY, "IS WITHIN ME NOW"

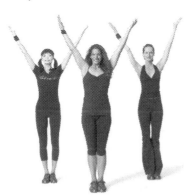

Step your feet back together. Extend your arms overhead in a V-position, your fingers wide, and look up to the sky.

GRATITUDE

SAY, "FOR MY LIFE"

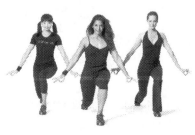

Step back to a rear lunge with your right foot. Extend your arms down and out by your sides, your palms facing down. Join your thumbs and index fingers to form the chin mudra, which is a hand gesture.

GRATITUDE TO OTHERS

SAY, "ALL OTHERS"

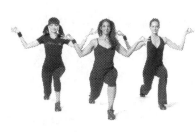

Hold the rear lunge. Rotate your hands back with your palms facing upward, your elbows slightly bent and by your sides. Your hands remain in the chin mudra.

GRATITUDE TO SELF

SAY, "AND MYSELF."

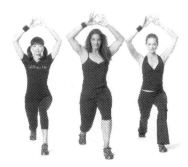

Remain in the rear lunge. Extend your arms overhead, keeping your elbows slightly bent. With your hands in the chin mudra, join your thumbs with your index fingers above your head to create the crown mudra.

ACCEPTANCE

SAY, "I ACCEPT"

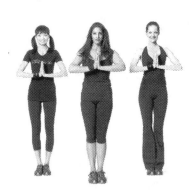

Step up to a standing balance, bending your right knee. With your hands in fists, cross your arms overhead. Bring your feet together. Bring your arms down and press your palms together in the Prayer position in front of your heart.

LOVE

SAY, "AND I LOVE"

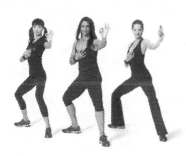

Step diagonally to the back with the right foot into the Warrior stance. Create two circles by touching your thumbs and index fingers (this is a slight variation of the chin mudra). Place your right palm over your heart, extend your left arm forward, and gaze through the circle as through a keyhole.

Notice the hand gesture: One hand on your heart and one in front of your eye. You are declaring that you are willing to see yourself and others through the eyes of love. See if you can focus through the hole between your thumb and index finger. This will work your inner thighs if you go down nice and low. Also try this extra tip: while you are in the pose, squeeze your heels toward each other, and you will feel your inner thighs working. This will also help eliminate pressure on your knees. Feel the presence of love. Remember, it is all about choosing it. It is there!

COMPASSION

SAY, "MYSELF"

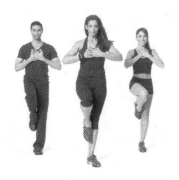

Step up to a single-leg balance with your right knee bent. Place your palms over your heart.

WARRIOR

SAY, "EXACTLY"

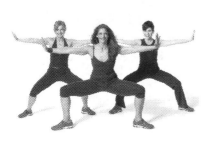

Step to the right in the Warrior stance with your arms extended straight to either side, your hands flexed back.

READY

SAY, "AS I AM."

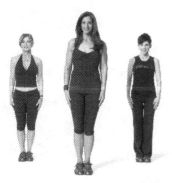

Step your right foot back to feet together. Stand tall, your feet together, your arms by your sides, and look straight ahead.

SERIES BREAKDOWN

Say, "All I need is within me now" (EMBRACE / POSITIVE EXPECTATION)

- "All I need"—EMBRACE. Give yourself a big hug.
- "is within me now"—POSITIVE EXPECTATION. Your arms extend in a "V" overhead.

Combine the two moves on the right side only for one minute, then on the left side only for one minute, then alternate right and left for one minute.

Say, "For my life, all others, and myself, I accept" (GRATI-TUDE / PEACE)

- "For my life"—GRATITUDE. Rear lunge, your hands face down, your thumbs and index fingers touch.
- "All others"—GRATITUDE. Remain in rear lunge, rotate your hands up, your thumbs and index fingers touch.
- "And myself"—GRATITUDE. Remain in rear lunge, your middle fingers, thumbs, and index fingers join overhead.
- "I accept"—ACCEPTANCE. Step up to a single-leg balance, your hands in the Prayer position over your heart.

Combine these moves on the right side only for one minute, then on the left side only for one minute, then alternate right and left for one minute.

Now run through the series from the top:

- "All I need is within me now" (EMBRACE / POSITIVE EXPECTATION)
- "For my life, all others, and myself, I accept" (GRATITUDE / ACCEPTANCE)

First run through 8 times on the right side, then 8 times on the left, then alternate 8 times right and left.

Say, "And I love myself exactly as I am" (LOVE / COMPAS-SION / WARRIOR READY)

- "And I love"—LOVE. Step back to the diagonal and look through the circle of your extended fingers as through a keyhole.
- "Myself"—COMPASSION. Step up to a single-leg balance, your hands crossed over your heart.
- "exactly as I am"—READY. Your feet together, your hands by your side.

Combine these three moves on the right side only for one minute, then on the left side only for one minute, then alternate right and left for one minute.

Now run through the entire series from the top. First run through the series 8 times on the right side, then 8 times on the left, then alternate 8 times right and left.

- "All I need is within me now" (EMBRACE / POSITIVE EXPECTATION)
- "For my life, all others, and myself, I accept" (GRATITUDE / ACCEPTANCE)
- "And I love myself exactly as I am" (LOVE / COMPASSION / WARRIOR READY)

CHAPTER CHECKLIST
i Will . . .

❋ Practice looking in the mirror and saying, "I love and accept myself as I am."

❋ Stop focusing on my flaws and dwelling on what I cannot change. Instead, I will focus my energy on changing what I can.

❋ Love instead of hate: myself, my body, my life.

principle seven

TAP INTO THE POWER
OF THE PRESENT

---

ongratulations! The last of these 7 Principles is the beginning of a whole new you! You now know new ways to think, to take action, to react to your feelings, to deal with disappointment, to honor and love yourself. But here comes the biggest challenge you will face: What will you do with what you've learned? How will you put these principles into play in your life? Will the end of this book be the end of your commitment to a better you—or will you keep it going, keep striving for more of what you know you want and deserve?

We've talked a great deal about "knowing yourself." So now, I'd like you to be honest and answer the following:

* Are you someone who always finishes what you start?
* Are you easily inspired into action—but that fire burns out quickly?
* Do you tend to *almost* succeed and then give up right before you are about to have a big breakthrough?
* Do you always finish the books you begin reading?

* Do you find it easy to make changes?
* Do you become easily frustrated if something is challenging?
* Do you enjoy trying new things?
* Do you need to see results to believe something is working?
* Do you keep promises you make to yourself and others?
* Do you get tired of/bored with routine?

Look over your answers. Then realize this: how you do *anything* is going to be how you do *everything*. And most often, how you used to do things is how you will continue to do them. Unless . . . you don't! My goal has been to get you to do things differently than you have before. To be different than you were in some way, any way. You haven't been happy with the direction your life has been going in (which is why you picked up this book in the first place!). The only way to achieve a future that doesn't resemble a version of your past is to change the present.

Make Today Count, One Day at a Time

Your life is happening right now. If you can put 90 percent of your attention on today ("What can I do today? What is important for me today? How can I feel good today?"), you will succeed in creating a future different from your past. Have you ever been able to stick to your promises *for one day*? Have you been able to make powerful, positive choices *for one day*? Of course you have! Well, right there is evidence that you *can* do it. When you live one day at a time, take your attention off the person you were and place your focus on the powerful present moment, where you *can* make a new choice, you have the ability to be anyone you want to be. As soon as you make that new choice—as soon as you say, "Yes! I can change!" instead of "No, I can't"—you will feel the change begin to happen.

Try not to overthink or project too far into the future. If you approach a situation with a sense of doom or dread, it's not going to motivate you to stick with it. You think, "Oh no! I have to exercise for the rest of my life!" or "I have to give up sugar for the next forty years," and you wonder why you're scared? Your life is happening *now*. You can feel good only *now*. You can imagine feeling good in the future or remember feeling good in the past, but your goal is simply to deal with this very day, this very minute. Don't worry what tomorrow will bring. It will bring a new opportunity for you to take an action that is either with or against your goal.

One of the most powerful phrases in a 12-step program is the reminder that you have to take it only "one day at a time." This concept has helped millions of people get through the toughest of times. Every time I would complain, "You mean I can't *ever* have sugar again? What about my wedding cake? What about my birthday, what about . . . ?" my sponsor would reply, "Just today. Just don't have that cake or that sugar *today*." I would breathe a sigh of relief! "Today" was totally doable. I could muster the strength and courage I needed for twenty-four hours. I wasn't committing just yet to a lifetime of sugar-free existence! But with every new day of making that "no-sugar" choice, it became easier; the dread disappeared.

In *The Molecules of Emotion*, Candace Pert states, "The more you engage in any type of emotion or behavior, the greater your desire for it will be." This can work to your advantage or disadvantage. If you have been engaging in a lot of negative behavior, it will be easier and easier to continue that behavior. That's what makes change so difficult. But once you put into action some positive behavior, it becomes easier and easier to live a healthy and happy life.

Pert explains that emotions are carried around our bodies by peptides (informational substances) that change the chemical properties of every cell in our bodies as they bind to receptor sites located on the cell. Translation: Your body is replacing worn-out or damaged cells all the time. An estimated 300 million cell divisions occur every minute to replace cells that die, and new cells are created according to what you think and feel. Stop and read that last line again! If you feel depressed for an hour, you've produced approximately 18 billion new cells that have more receptors calling out for depressed-type peptides and fewer calling out for gratitude, love, appreciation, or joy. So if you spend an hour feeling good, if you improve your mood even 20 percent of the time, your body will become more susceptible to that emotion. You will "crave" happiness, health, and vitality—and you will have a much easier time "feeding" that craving with positive new choices.

ᑎo ᖇegrets

Have you ever looked at a picture of yourself from years ago and wondered, "Oh, what did I have to complain about back then? If only I looked that good now!" Maybe if you had done this or done that, things would be different? Let it go! You can stop living in the past and "what if-ing" yourself. A fulfilling goal is to live with no regrets. Regret is not an emotion that feels good, so turn your regrets into powerful motivators and make a commitment to yourself to learn from your past.

What can you learn? Not to repeat the same thing; to find a way to be grateful where you are right now. You can't go back in time, but you can slow down the feeling of losing time by paying attention to what you are doing now, how you are living now, and making choices that you are proud of. The practice of *mindfulness*—bringing conscious awareness to your moment-by-moment choices—is the only way to change the course of your life.

When I have a room full of students and they are sweating and working hard, I purposely introduce an exercise that will push them to a point of challenging discomfort—and then ask them to do more. After 20 minutes of intense cardio, I have them drop and do 30 repetitions of the exercise I call "Determination." The response the first time I do this is usually moans and groans: "No way! You've got to be kidding!" But I'm not kidding, and there's a method to my madness! I say, "Use your warrior spirit here! Stop whining and just do what you can do." Think about those words: "Do what you can do." Nothing more, just what you are able to handle, whether it's 1 repetition or 50—I want you to push yourself a little extra to do what you can do.

And guess what? Not only does the majority of the class easily complete the exercise at that moment, but they walk out of that room with a newfound sense of pride and self-confidence. It is the most empowering feeling of growth; when you get yourself to the edge of your comfort zone and you surpass it, you feel alive. When you do less than you are able to do, you miss out on the rush and the incredible sense of accomplishment. Eventually, when I tell that class, "Gimme ten more!" instead of whining, they learn to respond, "Bring it on!" This doesn't have to apply just to exercise. Do what you can do *today*. Every little bit counts.

Never Give Up

When I first began teaching fitness classes, I was in heaven. I was sure I had found my calling. I was about eighteen years old and in my freshman year of college at San Jose State University, and I was unsure about what I wanted to study or do with the rest of my life. What I did know was that everything in my life had to fit in around my teaching schedule. That sure spoke volumes; it was the most important thing to me, and I couldn't even dream of doing anything else. Of course, there were plenty of naysayers. "Patricia," they scoffed, "this sort of career depends on your body. How long are you *really* going to be able to do this? *Then* what are you going to do?" I wasn't sure. I didn't have the answers. All I knew was that I wouldn't give it up; I would follow my heart and my passion and trust that it would take me someplace I couldn't even imagine. When something feels that life-enhancing, when it makes you happy, when you become stronger and more alive by living it, then it will always lead you in the right direction.

I have had the great pleasure of being at the forefront of the fitness industry boom, but it took an incredible amount of faith to take one day at a time and trust that the next opportunity would reveal itself. My greatest success is that my life has been consistently improving, my health has been consistently improving, and my level of happiness has been consistently growing. I have tried many things and I have failed at many things, but through it all I have developed a clearer and clearer picture of how I want to live and who I want to be. You may not always know the way in your own life, but if you keep the dream alive and you want your life to improve, then day by day it will. It is up to you, so . . .

❋ Never give up your dream.
❋ Never give up on yourself.

- ❋ Never give up on improving with age.
- ❋ Never give up on knowing that life is meant to be lived any way we choose to live it.
- ❋ Never give up your power by blaming others, your past, or circumstances in your life for your unhappiness.
- ❋ Believe that you are in the right place, this is the right time, and you can do it.
- ❋ Every success and every failure you have had is *exactly* what you needed at that time. They have all led you here, to where you're supposed to be. Without failure, we'd never know what success truly tastes like.

What Are You Waiting For?

One of my sisters is twelve years older than me, and for as long as I can remember she has had a weight problem. At the age of fifty, she made a decision to change her life. In less than two years she dropped 150 pounds. How did she do it? She finally felt the pain of being overweight and not living life. She had sessions with my life coach; she did the IntenSati workout along with other workouts; and she succeeded. Her only regret was not doing it sooner.

Procrastination is one of the most common causes of failure. Most of us keep putting off change and waiting for "the right moment." But there may never be that perfectly right time; the only moment there ever is is *now*. The only way any information is useful is if you put it into action. Start wherever you are, with whatever you can do. What is so powerfully important to remember is that the moment you just stop doing what you have been doing, you are already making a positive change.

Although you may not see any physical change in your body right away, what you will gain is much more important: inner strength. When you stop the momentum from going in the direction you don't want it to go in, that is quite an accomplishment. Recognize it and pat yourself on the back. When you buy a book like this one, it is a step in the right direction: You are keeping yourself in the game. You could read a trashy novel or a book on how to make desserts. Instead, you are reading this book, and the information in it is feeding you on a spiritual level. It is causing you to think differently.

How can you make a change that has an immediate impact?

❋ Do the exercises in this book; make them part of your life every single day. Don't put them off. Even if you do one exercise, even if you do one affirmation or assignment, you will continue moving in the direction you want to go in.

❋ When you are driving in a car and you are lost, what's the best thing you can do? Stop, so you don't get farther away from your desired destination! Stop complaining, stop doubting, stop hating yourself. All you have to do sometimes is *stop*! And when you stop complaining, what is left? When you stop doubting, what is available? When you stop hating yourself, what is possible?

❋ Get over the "all-or-nothing" mentality. Take off the pressure of having to "get it right" and instead just do it. You will never regret doing it, but you could (like my sister) regret not doing it sooner.

By now you have felt the greatness within you, whether it's just bubbling to the surface or overflowing out of every pore. You know what you can do, and you know how to do it. As you reach the end of these principles, the only homework assignment that remains is taking it to the next level. What will you do now? What new goals, challenges, dreams will you pursue? What questions will you ask yourself? How will you continue to grow and grasp for that brass ring, even after you have accomplished what you set out to accomplish?

You are blessed with everything you need to succeed at anything you want to succeed in. Your number one challenge will be overcoming your own limiting beliefs. There is simply no way around this challenge; the only way is to face it, to go through it,

---

WAKE UP A WARRIOR!

Before you get out of bed in the morning, after you turn off your alarm, lie there for five minutes or so and just imagine living the day as a warrior. How will you dress, think, eat, talk, and walk? Play the part out in your mind first.

I learned one of the most powerful lessons of my life when I was twelve years old. I had a life-threatening infection in the bone marrow of my left arm. The night before I was going to have surgery (and possibly have my arm amputated), my father came into the hospital after everyone had gone home and pulled up a chair next to my bed. He told me we were going to play a game. He told me to close my eyes and imagine an army of soldiers marching into my arm. Each one had a pick, a shovel, or a hose, and they were each coming to clean out the infection. One by one, we visualized each little soldier in his uniform doing his part. Then the group of soldiers marched out, one by one, taking the infection with them. The next group marched in to patch it up.

Miraculously, when the doctors came in the next morning, they found that the infection was gone. They had no idea how—but Dad and I did!

Practice using your imagination to see yourself marching through your day with ease, with courage, with enjoyment. For even just a few minutes before you get moving, see yourself eating well, working out, and moving through your day successfully. It's a small effort with big rewards. March on! 🔲

to deal with it and to know that what is on the other side is freedom. Peace of mind will come when you allow yourself to become who you are yearning to become. The discomfort and struggle are created in your mind when you don't believe in yourself—when your heart wants something but you lack the practice in getting there.

The way I see it, every ending is a beginning. Every day you get a new chance to do it better, to try again, to learn something new, and to improve how you are living. If you get the momentum going in a new direction, that momentum will carry you powerfully into a new future. There is nothing holding you back; there are no more excuses. So what will you do today? Reflect, sweat, challenge yourself, eat well, burn some calories, feel accomplished, learn, and grow. Are you ready? Are you a warrior?

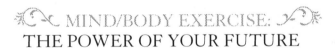

MIND/BODY EXERCISE:
THE POWER OF YOUR FUTURE

I am intended
To have all I desire.
I claim my power
And the truth sets me free.

As you put this all together, let each word match each pose. Repeat each move until you feel comfortable with it. At first you may not move smoothly, but that is a sign that you are learning. Don't give up. Your goal is to do this entire exercise without looking at the book. For an advanced workout, go through every chapter from the beginning and string all the exercises together. Memorize them. Practice them, and you will see how they begin to change you from the inside out. Enjoy the process!

CHOOSE

SAY, "I AM"

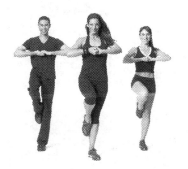

Take a single-leg balance, your right knee up. Bend your elbows, link your hands in front of your heart, and pull your hands apart to activate your upper back muscles.

INTENTION

SAY, "INTENDED"

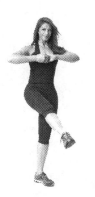

Remain in balance with your hands linked with intention, and straighten your right leg in front of you.

POSITIVE EXPECTATION

SAY, "TO HAVE ALL"

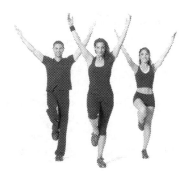

Now bend your knee back as you stay in a single-leg balance and extend your arms above your head in a V-position.

DESIRE

SAY, "I DESIRE."

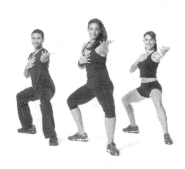

Step back in a Warrior stance with your right leg diagonally toward the back. Place your right palm over your heart and extend your left arm in front of you, your palm facing up to the sky.

CONFIDENCE

SAY, "I CLAIM"

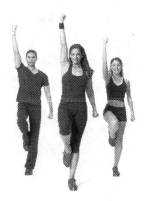

Again, step up to a single-leg balance with your right knee bent. With fists, extend your left arm down toward the ground and confidently extend your right arm over your head.

POWER

SAY, "MY POWER"

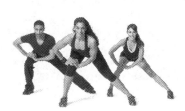

Step to the right in a deep, powerful lunge, keeping your back straight and your feet parallel. Place both hands on your right thigh for support.

COMPASSION

SAY, "AND THE TRUTH"

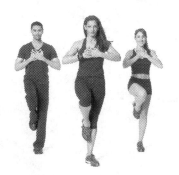

Step back to a single-leg balance, your right knee up and bent. Place your flattened palms on your chest.

STRENGTH

SAY, "SETS ME FREE."

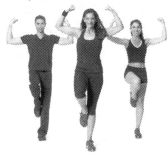

Stay in the single-leg balance. Make fists with your hands and circle your arms up and around until they are parallel with the floor in a double-biceps pose. Stand strong, keeping your heart open. Repeat all moves on the left side.

SERIES BREAKDOWN

Say, "I am intended" (CHOOSE / INTENTION)
- "I am"—CHOOSE. Stand in a single-leg balance and link hands in front of your heart.
- "intended"—INTENTION. Extend your leg.

Combine the two moves on the right side only for one minute, then on the left side only for one minute, then alternate right and left for one minute.

Say, "To have all I desire" (POSITIVE EXPECTATION / DESIRE)
- "To have all"—POSITIVE EXPECTATION. Extend your arms overhead in a V-position.
- "I desire"—DESIRE. Step diagonally toward the back, and extend one arm forward, palm up.

Combine these moves on the right side only for one minute, then on the left side only for one minute, then alternate right and left for one minute.

Now run through the series from the top:
- "I am intended" (CHOOSE / INTENTION)
- "To have all I desire" (POSITIVE EXPECTATION / DESIRE)

Run through 8 times on the right side, then 8 times on the left, then alternate 8 times right and left.

Say, "I claim my power" (CONFIDENCE / POWER)
- "I claim"—CONFIDENCE. Reach up high with one arm while in a single-leg balance.
- "my power"—POWER. Step up to a deep side lunge.

Combine these two moves on the right side only for one minute, then on the left side only for one minute, then alternate right and left for one minute.

Say "And the truth sets me free" (COMPASSION / STRENGTH)
- "And the truth"—COMPASSION. Remain in a single-leg balance, cross palms over your heart.
- "Sets me free"—STRENGTH. Circle your arms to a double-biceps curl.

Combine these two moves on the right side only for one minute, then on the left side only for one minute, then alternate right and left for one minute.

Now run through the series from the top:
- "I am intended" (CHOOSE / INTENTION)
- "To have all I desire" (POSITIVE EXPECTATION / DESIRE)
- "I claim my power" (CONFIDENCE / POWER)
- "And the truth sets me free" (COMPASSION / STRENGTH)

Run through 8 times on the right side, then 8 times on the left, then alternate 8 times right and left.

CHAPTER CHECKLIST
i Will . . .

❋ Stop procrastinating! Focus on feeling better *right now* . . . not tomorrow or the next day.

❋ Drop regrets about the past and worries about the future.

❋ Lie in bed for a few minutes after waking up every morning, mentally picturing myself going through the day successfully and with ease.

NOURISH THE NEW YOU

I know diets. I have been on dozens of them. I understand the allure: You want to believe that a "miracle diet" will give you fab abs overnight or shrink you three sizes smaller by the weekend. Most of them ask you to commit to an unsustainable (and undesirable) regime of deprivation and tasteless food. And when that is what you have to look forward to ("I'll never be able to stick to this!"), your fear of failure defeats you before you even begin.

But you're right about one thing: If you don't feel that the food plan is one you can embrace and follow your entire life, you won't be able to keep it going. Banish the fear factor in food. You shouldn't feel you are being punished or restricted or reined in. You are choosing what to eat and what not to eat. Everything you put into your mouth is honoring your commitment to yourself and your goal. So instead of adopting a diet that defeats your positive feelings about yourself, you are going to adopt a way to eat to thrive, not just survive.

Why do you suppose I placed this meal-plan section at the end of the book? Because this weight-loss program is different from all the others. I want you to give as much attention to your mental and physical health as you do to your nutritional health. It all works together as a team, but there is an order to things. What I have put together for you is a "food philosophy" that I have found made the biggest difference for me over the years. What I practice is a lifestyle, a long-term, life-enhancing way of living, which will have you continually evolving into a healthier and happier you. With this plan, you get to add to your life instead of take away.

I feel very passionate about this approach to weight loss because of my childhood. I grew up with a mother who dieted all her life in very extreme ways, and I witnessed firsthand her painful struggle. Her pain and battle kept increasing while her weight and her health continued to worsen. For a long time, I did many of the same things she did. I knew there had to be a better way that was healthier and long-lasting. For those of you who like a quick fix, you might not be thrilled at first; the weight is not going to melt off as it would on a crash diet. But you will get your quick fix in another way: you'll feel better as soon as you start. And the longer you stick to it, the longer you will reap the rewards.

My Weight-Loss Saga

For years, I tried the diet du jour; I went from being a vegetarian to eating a high-protein diet to a restricted-carb diet to a raw diet to fasts and supplements. I had had it. I was ready to let go of the "diet mentality." I decided to learn more about nutrition so I could feel better informed and make a decision about what was right for me. The first thing I did was find a nutritionist who had a similar philosophy. She believed in a nutritional plan that was a long-term lifestyle, instead of a nonmaintainable deprivation game. When I walked into her office, I felt such a sense of relief! She continually educated me and reminded me that the work we were doing together was not just about "losing" but also "gaining." I would be gaining a better, smarter, more fulfilling way to live.

Every time I had a photo shoot, a DVD shoot, or a special event, I took the last 10 pounds off in drastic ways (of course, I always gained it back, which is why I was always trying to take it off again!). In a panic, I went to extremes: next-to-nothing calorie consumption, fasts, cleanses, diuretics, and excessive exercise. Then, in between this diet madness, I would feel I deserved more. I had been working so hard, training so hard, and depriving myself so much, I rationalized, "Hey, I should be able to eat what I want now!"

It was an endless cycle of abusing my body. What I really wanted was to live at the weight I was proud of and happy at without deprivation, without extreme measures of any kind. I called it "being normal." I just wanted to be normal! I wanted to eat, but not overeat. I wanted to be free from having food on my mind *all the time*. I wanted to enjoy my meals without guilt, and I especially wanted to be able to have a bite of a dessert and walk away or have one cookie and not fight with myself to keep my hands out of that cookie jar. I feared that eating "just one" would never be enough, so I would never buy anything too tempting. As a result, my apartment was filled with boring, tasteless foods that I would not want to overeat (or even eat at all!). No one ever got fat on broccoli and brussels sprouts, right?

I remember in my darkest times feeling so guilty about eating that I wouldn't eat in public places. I was a closet eater, because I had made food my enemy. I thought that no matter what I ate, it was too much. I felt like a slave to food, a victim of my fears and insecurity. To give a cookie all that power over you—that's just ridiculous!

Starting to Heal

My life coach, Lauren Zander, helped me make a promise to myself and build my power of keeping my word to myself. My nutritionist, Lisa Jubilee of Living Proof Nutrition/Fitness (www.livingproofnyc.com), designed for me a way of eating that has helped me have it all—minus the guilt. Lisa's program is what I recommend for you, because I love the way it takes into consideration so many issues for women today: an on-the-go lifestyle, a love of sweets, a desire to stay in a range of weight, and a commitment to a healthy lifestyle. I find it sane and supportive. But there are days, I won't lie to you, when I can't have "just one" treat; I slip up. So what? That's my new motto! I am succeeding much more than I fail, and what a blessing to have come this far. To no longer *literally* be afraid of food!

This approach will help you regain your power over food, instead of seeing yourself as powerless. You can train yourself to do anything, but you need a clear goal. You need to do a little trial and error, and you have to persevere. Remember, a little compassion and patience will go a long way. I strongly urge you to build your own support team. Find people who are living well and living the way you want to, and get them on your side, whether it means hiring a life coach or a nutritionist, joining a 12-step program (such as Overeaters Anonymous or GreySheeters Anonymous), or going to a weight-loss meeting—even if you have to put a group together on your own! And most important, make sure *you're* on your side! Stay true to your goals; practice all the principles you've learned in this book. Don't let anyone or anything discourage you. This time will be different. This time you will succeed. Why? Because you are already a different person, a stronger, healthier, happier person. The New You knows no defeat!

The Anti-Diet

The number one key to your success on your new Anti-Diet is changing your outlook about food overall. Food is an amazing thing. It has the potential to heal or kill. The two main issues are quality and quantity. With endless numbers of diet books on the market, it can all get very confusing and complicated. So many people ask me, "What should I eat?" I have been asking myself this question my entire life, and I have reached out to experts, gone to workshops, enrolled in nutrition classes, read numerous books, and experimented on myself. What I have narrowed it down to is this basic statement: "Eat good-quality food and have a good-quality life!" Really! Eating well doesn't have to be that complicated.

When you look at the average American diet, it is filled with fast foods, processed foods, additives, preservatives, chemicals, pesticides, hormones, and antibiotics—not what Mother Nature intended for us to be consuming. The average American diet is far from a good-quality diet. We can see it when we see the statistics of the rise of obesity, heart disease, diabetes, and other diet-related illnesses. A study by the Centers for Disease Control and Prevention found that diet and inactivity may soon overtake smoking as the leading cause of death in the United States.

Stop striving to be "skinny" and focus more on getting your body healthy, fit, and feeling great. Many people go to great lengths to try to lose weight and take their attention off the quality of the food they are eating. I have been there myself: I used to make a salad consisting of the lowest-calorie nonorganic vegetables I could find, sprinkled with (I know it sounds disgusting) Splenda and I Can't Believe It's Not Butter. All I cared about was losing weight—not how I was fueling my body. I was also endlessly chewing sugar-free gum to curb my cravings. Now I know that Splenda, sugar, and artificial sweeteners can actually *increase* your appetite.

The Concept of "Crowding Out"

The best diet is not a diet at all. It's a checklist of things you can indulge in—not a list of things you should be eliminating. I am going to give you lists of foods, and you are going to add as many of these foods to your diet as you can. Trust yourself. Notice how you feel. Enjoy your food and recognize that *the quality of your life deeply depends on the quality of your food*.

There are only so many hours in a day. Even if you consider yourself someone who eats *a lot*, there is only so much you can consume in twenty-four hours. If you make a commitment to eat foods packed with nutritional value, minerals, vitamins, and good, clean sources of protein, carbs, and fats *before* you impulsively reach for fast food, candy bars, or bags of chips, there simply will not be enough time in the day—or room in your stomach—for much of the other stuff.

"But, Patricia," you say, "I just can't live without chocolate" (or pizza, or cookies, or whatever your favorite comfort food is). Don't worry! This plan is about empowering you and removing your feelings of guilt and fear about food. So you're going to work the 90/10 plan: strive to eat well 90 percent of the time, and 10 percent of the time, eat whatever you want. For me, whenever I would binge on some dessert or sweet treat in the past, I would tell myself, "That's it! This is the last time!" And of course it wasn't. Why? Because the more you tell yourself you can't have something, the more you want it. On the 90/10 plan, you can have little treats—guilt-free! If you want to have birthday cake, go for it. If you want to have a slice of pizza, eat it without guilt. Then go back to eating the best food you can. You can even plan a once-a-week meal

Words of Wisdom

"Thou shouldst eat to live; not live to eat."—Socrates

where you are going to indulge in something you don't have all the time. Maybe it's pancakes for breakfast on Sunday. It could be your Saturday-night steak night. It might be your Sunday Mexican food brunch. Whatever works for you and makes you happy.

Getting Started

Everybody—and every body—is different. Some people like to go cold turkey and make drastic changes all at once. Others need the slow but steady approach. You have to choose what works best for you, but either way, remember to take it one day at a time. You are building new habits, and as you do, the old habits will begin to lose their grip on you.

Take your attention off calorie counting and keep your attention on feeling good, eating whole foods, cutting down on processed foods, and exercising more. If you get too caught up in calorie counting, you will be feeding your "diet" habit instead of your "living" habit. I know that for some of you that might be a hard habit to break, but remember, if you want to change the outcome, you are going to have to change your actions. Your overall goal is to focus on high-quality, low-calorie foods. I promise, you will not starve! In fact, you will be eating *more* food, getting more nutrients, and feeling more satisfied on fewer calories. Great food will change your life, but you have to eat it!

Choose foods from all the following lists, and incorporate them into your daily eating plans (you'll find three samples of mine on pages 164–65). Remember, variety is the name of the game. Be adventurous! Try new things, and when you do, you will train your palate. The body is incredible and will heal itself if you just give it what it needs. If you have been living on a diet of fast food, meals on the go, protein bars, candy bars, coffee, soda, processed foods, and very little real food, your life and your health will drastically improve almost immediately. How's that for an incentive to get started right now?

Superfoods

GOJI BERRIES

You may have heard of these little bright-orange raisinlike fruits or have seen them popping up in your grocery store and wondered what all the excitement was about. Well, these little superstars are known to enhance your stamina, strength, longevity, and sexual energy. They also boost the immune system. Eat a handful a day! You can buy them online at www.sunfood .com, at your health food store, or at grocery stores like Whole Foods.

RAW CACAO

This is not the chocolate you find in a Hershey's candy bar; I'm talking raw chocolate powder or nibs. In ancient times it was known as not only a food but a potent medicine. It contains 314 percent of the U.S. RDA of iron per ounce, improves mental performance, increases longevity, may lower blood pressure, and is rich in antioxidants. I use raw cacao in so many different ways: I put a tablespoon of it in my morning oatmeal, sprinkle it on fruit, or mix it with goji berries and add cashews to make a trail mix. You can buy them in your health food store or online at www.sun food.com or www.channelingchocolate.com. Eat without guilt!

HEMP SEED

This is one of nature's richest sources of protein. It contains all the essential amino acids and essential fatty acids necessary to maintain a super-fit, super-healthy super life! Sprinkle it on salads, drop it in a smoothie, or grab a handful on the go! Buy it in the health food store or online at www.sunfood.com.

COCONUT OR COCONUT OIL

Coconut oil cuts your appetite, enabling you to go for hours feeling satisfied. Eating fresh coconut, drinking coconut water, or adding coconut oil to your diet will actually increase your metabolic rate and help you lose weight. I add a tablespoon of it to my oatmeal or my smoothies, and I also use it for salad dressing.

FLAXSEEDS

Flaxseeds are very high in omega-3 essential fatty acids—the good fat. They are known to lower cholesterol, stabilize blood sugar, lower the risk of breast, prostate, and colon cancer, and reduce the inflammation of arthritis. Buy ground flaxseed and add 1 to 2 teaspoons a day to your salads, shakes, cereal, yogurt, or any other food you want.

PUMPKIN SEEDS

You definitely want to add these super satisfying seeds to your list of YES foods. They naturally provide you with B vitamins, plus many minerals and essential fatty oils. Pumpkin seeds are also an aphrodisiac. Just a handful a day will help keep you feeling great.

RADISHES

These little spicy round balls of super nutrition should be added to your salads or as a midday snack with some cucumbers and tomato. They are great kidney cleansers, they decrease water retention, and they improve elimination. They are the highest vegetable sources of vitamin C.

AGAVE NECTAR

This is a great replacement for sugar and artificial sweeteners. You can pour it on oatmeal or in smoothies, use it for cooking, or even add it to salad dressing. Its sweetness comes primarily from a complex form of fructose called inulin, found naturally in fruits and vegetables. The carbohydrate in agave nectar has a low glycemic index, so you get the sweet taste without a sugar rush. You can find it online at www.sunfood.com or at your health food store.

Mood-Boosting Foods

Perfect to get you going in the morning or as an antidote for the afternoon blahs:

Apples	Mango
Bananas	Melons
Blackberries	Oranges
Blueberries	Papaya
Cantaloupe	Peaches
Coconut, fresh	Pears
Dark chocolate	Raspberries
Frozen acai berries	Raw cacao nibs
Goji berries	Strawberries

Power Foods

Try adding at least 3 cups from this list daily. Be adventurous. Try something new every day. Eat them raw, steamed, sautéed, juiced, all together, or one at a time. Eat them any time of day, all day, any day!

Arugula
Asparagus
Bell peppers
Bok choy
Broccoli
Brussels sprouts
Carrots
Cauliflower
Celery
Collard greens
Cucumber
Fennel
Kale

Lettuce
Sea vegetables (arama, dulse, hijiki, wakane)
Seaweed, vegetable sushi rolls wrapped in seaweed
Snow peas
Spinach
Sprouts, all types
Swiss chard
Water chestnuts
Watercress
Zucchini

Satisfying Snacks

These will help you feel IntenSati-sfied and happy! They are great on-the-go snacks, additions to your meals, airplane food, taxi food, road trip snacks, ballpark treats, movie snacks, dog-walking pocket food, and hiking energy boosters! Just eat them in moderation (you can squeeze in one or two a day and squeeze out the cookies, chips, candy bars, peanuts, buttered popcorn, super-size sodas, etc.). Buy them at any health food store, Whole Foods, or online. Feed them to your kids, too!

Raw cashews
Raw almonds
Walnuts
Pumpkin seeds
Air-popped popcorn
Baked chips of any kind
Vegetable chips
Multigrain tortilla chips
Organic dark chocolate
    bars
Kind nut bars
Lara bars
Organic pretzels
Organic dried mulberries

Avocados
Hard-boiled eggs
Flaxseed crackers
Greek or plain yogurt with
    fruit or agave
Hummus
Single stick of
    string cheese
Steamed edamame
Himilania dark chocolate–
    covered goji berries
    (Whole Foods Stores)
Raw crunch energy bar
    (www.sunfood.com)

Warrior Builders

Make these your protein choices. Eat a palm-sized serving once or twice a day. Make sure you pick the best quality. Buy grass-fed, free-range, organic, fresh items.

Omega-3 eggs
Chicken breast
Turkey
Salmon
Tuna
Soybeans
Tempeh
Mussels

Halibut
Scallops
Sole
Shrimp
Hummus
Raw almond butter
Raw cashew butter
Quinoa

Good Fats

Fats don't *make* you fat; they give you energy. But they have to be the *right kind* of fat. Good fat boosts your fat-burning capabilities and helps you feel full longer. These fats will cut your appetite and increase your health.

Extra-virgin olive oil (2 tablespoons)

Avocado

Pumpkin seeds (handful)

Cashews (10–16)

Sesame seeds (1 tablespoon)

Almonds (10–15)

Flaxseeds and flaxseed oil (2 tablespoons)

Omega-3 fats (found in wild fish, especially salmon, or a supplement)

Coconut oil (1–4 tablespoons)

Macadamia nut oil

Putting It All Together

To start, try the following plan:

Pick 2 mood-boosting foods (fruit) (page 160)

Pick 6 power foods (carbohydrates) (page 161)

Pick 2 warrior builders (protein) (page 162)

Pick 2 cut-your-appetite foods (good fats) (page 163)

Pick 1 superfood (pages 158–60)

Pick 8 drinks to clear your mind and body (hydrating) (pages 166–67)

Pick once a week from Satisfying snacks (page 162)

Keep the foods in their natural form whenever possible. Steam, sauté, wok, dice up into salads, and pack a lunch or a snack bag whenever you can. Always have healthy snack options in your bag, office, or car. If you are on the go a lot, make it easy for yourself. When you have great food handy, you will reach for it before you get too hungry and reach for something worse.

My Anti-Diet lists don't, of course, include every food that is good for you. But once you start thinking about these foods, you'll have good-quality food on your mind, and you'll be on the lookout for more foods to add to your Anti-Diet. The key is to keep yourself satisfied. The more you eat the highly nutritious stuff, the easier and easier it will get!

Patricia's Sample Eating Plan

Here are a few days from my food diary. Use this to inspire you as you start your Anti-Diet!

DAY 1 (AVERAGE DAY)

BREAKFAST: Oatmeal topped with hemp seeds, agave, blueberries

SNACK: Vegetable juice (celery, parsley, carrot, ginger)

LUNCH: Salad (leafy greens, radishes, cucumbers, tomatoes, sprouts, water chestnuts, cauliflower, kidney beans, pumpkin seeds). Dressing: olive oil, a squeeze of lemon, a pinch of salt, and red chili pepper flakes

SNACK: Superfood smoothie (1 cup frozen mixed berries, 2 tablespoons raw cocoa powder or nibs, handful of goji berries, 2 tablespoons agave, water, and ice)

DINNER: Large bowl vegetable soup; 1 cup brown rice

DAY 2 (ON-THE-GO DAY)

BREAKFAST: Greek nonfat yogurt; cup of blueberries; 2 tablespoons ground flaxseed; green tea

SNACK: Apple; 10–15 raw almonds

LUNCH: Sprouted-grain tortilla wrap with chicken breast, tomato, avocado, salsa, bell pepper, sprouts, arugula

SNACK: Dark chocolate or raw chocolate square; hot raspberry tea

DINNER: Fennel and tomato salad with olive oil, mustard, and lemon dressing; grilled salmon; steamed kale

DAY 3 (WEEKEND)

BREAKFAST: Omega-3 egg scramble: 3 egg whites and 1 egg mixed with chopped tomato, spinach, bell peppers, asparagus, and avocado; 2 pieces whole grain sprouted bread; green tea

LUNCH: 1 cup brown rice, grilled vegetables; green salad with a variety of raw vegetables and tahini dressing

SNACK: Nonfat Greek yogurt sprinkled with sliced almonds and agave sweetener

DINNER: Cucumber and tomato salad; baked halibut; baked sweet potato; sautéed brussels sprouts

More Anti-Diet Tips to Add to Your Practice

HYDRATE! Our body is made up of mostly water. We need to make sure it is fully hydrated. Many people don't drink enough water and instead reach for soda, coffee, milk, alcohol, or juices as a replacement, but nothing can replace water. It helps cut your appetite, it flushes out toxins, it helps clear your skin, it can help relieve headaches, increase your energy, clear your mind, and make you feel alive. When you are dehydrated, your body does not work as efficiently. Often when you feel hunger pangs, you are just thirsty. If you make it a habit every day to drink 8 glasses of water or 6 glasses of water and 2 of another choice from the list below, you will not be able to eat as much. The water will fill you up and regulate your system. This is absolutely one of the best things you can do for yourself. Get into the habit of drinking water, or one of the drinks from this list before you go for anything else!

If you have not been drinking water regularly, this list alone will make a huge difference for you. If 6 to 8 glasses is too much for you to handle in the beginning, start with 4 and work your way up. How can you fit it all in? Carry it with you. Fill a reusable water bottle. You can buy a 32-ounce bottle and fill it twice a day to keep track. Squeeze some lemon in there and go! Start the day with a cup or two of hot water with lemon, and you are good to go!

Drinks to Clear Your Mind and Body

Great-quality water: filtered, bottled, or spring
Hot water with lemon (detoxifies)
Filtered water with lemon juice, cayenne pepper, and
   agave
Ginseng tea (energy and metabolism booster)

Dandelion root tea (detoxifies)
Raspberry tea (great for women)
Yerba maté (coffee replacement)
Rooibos tea (helps increase energy and cut appetite)
Peppermint tea (soothes an upset stomach)
Licorice tea (satisfies a sweet tooth!)

SATISFY YOUR SWEET TOOTH, NATURALLY. Nowadays there are some great sugar replacements for you to use instead of regular sugar and artificial sweeteners. Sugar is the one thing all experts in the field of health and nutrition urge us to cut from our diet or drastically reduce. According to Dr. Mark Hyman, M.D., the author of *Ultra Metabolism*, "the average person eats about 180 lbs. of sugar a year, or about ½ pound per person per day. When you eat sugar, you unconsciously start a vicious cycle of cravings, increased insulin production, increased appetite, more sugar intake, and more insulin production until you are in a cycle of cravings, bingeing and crashing all day long."

So what can we do? First of all, if you are adding power, super, mood-enhancing, appetite-cutting, and satisfying foods to your diet, you will be eliminating sugar. But if you want to add sweetener to your tea, yogurt, oatmeal, or superfood shake, choose from these:

Raw agave
Yacon root (similar to maple syrup)
Stevia (natural and very sweet; carry this in your bag and
add it instead of sugar whenever you need to)

CHOOSE WHOLE FOODS. These are foods the way Mother Nature intended them; they are in their natural state. They contain no added sugar, salt, fat, or synthetic preservatives, flavorings, or colorings. And when you take pleasure in feeding yourself this type of high-quality, organic, live, unprocessed, *real* food, you will never have to count calories again. Your body, if given half a chance, will always find its way back to its natural healthy, happy state.

FILL UP ON FRUIT. Most experts recommend two servings of fruit a day. But let's keep this simple and use common sense: Choose fruit over doughnuts, cookies, ice cream, bagels, cereal bars, sugary cereals, candy, or any fake food. Use fiber-packed fruit to satisfy your sweet tooth and keep you full. There are so many fruits to choose from, and, yes, some are better than others. Did you know that avocado, cucumber, and tomatoes are all fruits? Buy organic fruits when you can. Yes, they are more expensive, but they are free of pesticides. Your goal is to avoid putting any unnatural things into your body.

GO FOR GREENS. Vegetables have something you can get only from plant-based food: phytonutrients. Phytonutrients act as antioxidants, cancer inhibitors, and immune system boosters, and they reduce genetic damage due to pollution and environmental toxins. Vegetables that are rich in color are the most powerful! Eat your veggies as naturally as you can (I prefer raw over cooked). Try them in many ways. Slice them, dice them, steam them, sauté them. Wok them, mix them all up, and enjoy them with your whole heart and soul, knowing that every bite is a little gift to improve your life.

CONSUME SOME CARBS. I know for some people *carbs* is a scary word. But I'm talking about *good* carbs: fruits, vegetables, legumes, whole grains. If you can pick it, dig it out of the ground, or take it off a tree, you can eat it! Keep them fresh, simple, and as close to their natural state as possible. Cut out or dramatically reduce refined and highly processed carbs, white flour, breads, pasta, sugary junk food, and soda. Those are the carbs that will pack on the pounds.

DON'T FEAR FAT. Eating the right fats will help you feel satisfied. Fat is also essential for your skin, hair, joints, appetite control, and healing. It slows down the digestive process so the body has more time to absorb nutrients and helps keep your energy up. The fat-soluble vitamins, A, D, E, and K, can be absorbed only when fat is present.

Most of us don't have enough omega-3 fat in our diet. Health food stores now sell oil containing it as a supplement just in case you can't get it into your diet naturally. Make it a point to add fish, flaxseeds, flax oil, nuts, pumpkin seeds, and hemp seeds to your diet to increase your levels of this essential fat. Monounsaturated fats are also good for you (and have even been found to help reduce belly fat, according to a recent *Prevention* magazine study). You can get monounsaturated fat from avocados, hazelnuts, Brazil nuts, cashews, extra virgin olive oil, sesame seeds, and pumpkin seeds.

Try to reduce your intake of saturated fat—this is the kind of fat found mainly in animal products, red meat, and whole-milk dairy products like ice cream, butter, and cheese. Also carefully read labels and avoid palm kernel oil, cocoa butter, and palm oil. These oils are found in many products like coffee creamers, cookies, and processed junk food. You should also avoid trans fats and hydrogenated or partially hydrogenated fats. These man-made fats are used in processed foods to prolong shelf life. Trans fats are concentrated in margarine, solid vegetable shortening, and processed foods like cookies, chips, cakes, and pies.

PICK THE RIGHT PROTEINS. There are many sources of protein besides your typical steak, hamburger, turkey, or chicken. Think of animal protein as a side dish or a garnish on your plate instead of the main attraction. If you love to eat meat, reduce the amount you have to about a fist-size portion. Also, if you are a meat lover, please look for the best quality of meat you can find. There is a huge difference between grass-fed organic (the animal is fed grass and has not been injected with hormones or antibiotics) and feedlot (the animal is fed grain, especially corn, and is injected with hormones to fatten it up quickly). Organic meat is lower in fat and artery-clogging saturated fat and higher in omega-3s. Consider other ways to get your protein, such as seeds, nuts, and beans.

PATRICIA MORENO

CHAPTER CHECKLIST

i will . . .

❋ Read over the list of foods in this chapter and make a shopping list of all the foods I want to buy.

❋ Look for organic, free-range, grass-fed, high-quality foods.

❋ Remove all products from my kitchen that have trans fats, hydrogenated fats, partially hydrogenated fats, high-fructose corn syrup, MSG, or sugar of any kind listed as one of the first five ingredients.

THE INTENSATI
WORKOUT

$\mathcal{N}$ow that you've built your vocabulary and gotten your mind and your intentions strong, you're ready to leap into a full IntenSati workout! Take a moment to be still and focus on your intention. Take a moment of gratitude for the strength you already have. These simple actions will move you into a more powerful state of mind than if you were to just jump into your workout, because they help you to stop, value, and appreciate what you are about to do. You can do the workout as a whole, flowing from one exercise into the next, or choose specific exercises when you need them (for example, when you're starving, when you're tired, or when you're tempted).

Begin every workout with the warm-up from Principle 1: "Every day, in a very true way, I co-create my reality. As above, so below. This is what I know." Then pause for a minute with your hands at your heart and your eyes closed. Take a few deep breaths and set your intention for your workout. It may be something as simple as "Today I intend to feel better" or "I intend to shift my mood." When you clarify what you want and you intend it, you put your power behind your actions, and that is when great things happen! Remember that this workout is called IntenSati: *mindful intending.* The feeling of empowerment will rise within you every time you make a decision to change.

Read through all the affirmations before beginning your workout, and when you find one that inspires you, do that one. What makes this so powerful is the combination of the action and the affirmations. You will embody the words even if they don't feel true for you now. The more you embody the movements, the more the words will be in your body, heart, and mind, and you *will* become who you want to become.

It takes courage to do this workout. Remember, it's easy to be a pessimist. When you tell yourself that exercise won't make a difference, it gets you off the hook for having to take action. But when you develop an optimistic outlook and hold yourself accountable for your actions, you are cultivating the mental and physical attributes of an achiever.

The more often you do the workouts, the more beneficial they will be. You have to invest your time and energy in them for them to create a significant change in your body and your mind. Doing any workout once or twice will never be effective in giving you long-lasting results. How many times a week should you do it? And how many reps should you do during each workout? It depends on what you have been doing and what results you are committed to achieving. A few guidelines:

1. If you are a beginner, work out for 30 minutes per session. Work on one series at a time. Stick to one series for 30 days. Learn it. Memorize it. Get it into your body and mind so you don't have to look at the book to follow along. Getting to that point is a very impressive accomplishment, and it will take dedication to get there without giving up. But when you learn it and memorize it, you

will not only get into shape, you will also build your commitment to yourself. Every small accomplishment is a great victory to be celebrated. Twice a week is very good; three times a week is better. If you do these workouts four or five times a week, that is excellent.

2. How long should each workout be? If your goal is weight loss and mental empowerment, a minimum of 30 minutes per session is suggested. You can work up to one hour per session by adding together the warm-up, an upper-body series, and a lower-body series. You will get what you put into it. If you put 100 percent into it, you will get 100 percent improvement.

3. Consistency will be your greatest accomplishment! Training yourself to feel good, to improve your state of mind, your health, and your body can all be accomplished at once by doing these exercises. This is the ultimate mind/body workout—in one session you can get everything!

I have broken down each affirmation so that you can see what action your body is doing while you are saying the words. If you are a musical person, the counts may be helpful for you. Each count is like one beat of music. This is to help you find the rhythm of each series. It should sound almost as if you are singing lyrics to a song.

> ### Words to live by
> Today I challenge myself
> to reach for something better.

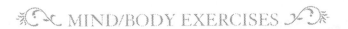

Exercise 1.

WHEN YOU ARE DOUBTING YOURSELF

Yes!
This I must achieve.
I will not stop
Until I succeed.
I am inspired now.
I am strong enough.
I am never giving up!

When you say these words, keep your attention on your intention. What is it that you must achieve? When you have plenty of reasons why you want to achieve your goals and you are committed to your success, you are unstoppable. Imagine the confidence you will build up in yourself after a few days of embodying this series!

COMMITMENT

SAY "YES!" EVERY TIME
THE LEFT ARM EXTENDS TO THE SKY

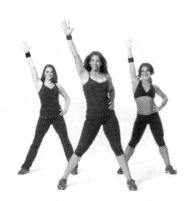

Stand with your feet more than shoulder width apart. Reach your right arm straight up over your head while slightly bending your right knee. Keep your left arm bent at your side. Both palms are facing forward.

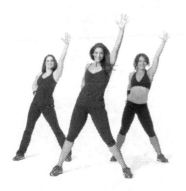

Now switch your arms, reaching your left arm straight up over your head while slightly bending your left knee. Keep your right arm bent by your side. Both palms are facing forward.

When you make your success a must, you will find a way! It takes courage to declare that you will succeed, no matter what! If you doubt you will succeed, you won't; if you choose to believe you will succeed, you will. Have the courage to believe in yourself.

DESIRE

SAY, "THIS I MUST ACHIEVE."

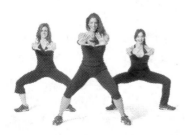

Assume the Warrior stance. Your hands are in front of you, with your thumbs and index fingers touching to create a triangle in front of your heart.

Remain in the Warrior stance. Keeping the triangle mudra with your hands, passionately extend your arms from your heart center.

Repeat out loud, "This I must achieve," for one minute.

Try to get yourself to the point where your arms are burning. Put as much fire into the motion as you can. Don't stop until you are sure you can't do any more. Practice getting to the point of failure.

Rhythm check: 4 counts
- ■ "This"—extend arms out and in
- ■ "I must"—extend arms out and in
- ■ "Achieve"—extend arms out and in 2 times

Run through for one minute:
- ■ "Yes"—4 counts (say "yes" out loud 2 times)
- ■ "This I must achieve"—4 counts

VICTORY

SAY, "I WILL NOT STOP"

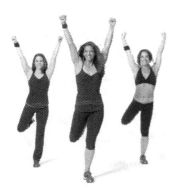

Jog in place and hold your arms up for 4 counts. When doing the action for one minute, raise your arms. Repeat out loud, "I will not stop" every time you speak out loud, and jog your arms by your sides for 4 counts.

Think of yourself crossing a finish line. Imagine you're the first one breaking through the tape. Feel the power of your victory before you even get there. See it, feel it, own it, and it will be yours!

FAITH

SAY, "UNTIL I SUCCEED."

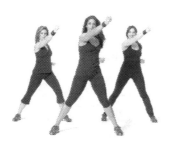

Stand with your feet hip width apart. Bend your elbows with your fists at either side of your chin. Powerfully punch your right fist up and diagonally across your body, allowing your torso to rotate to the left.

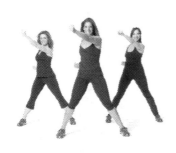

Bring your right fist back beside your chin and now powerfully punch your left fist up and diagonally across your body, allowing your torso to rotate to the right. Keep your elbows close to your sides and bring both fists back to either side of your chin after each punch.

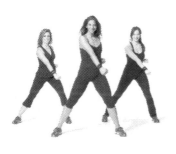

With your knees bent, powerfully punch your right fist down and diagonally across your body, allowing your torso to rotate to the left again. Make sure to keep your back straight and your abs in as you punch down.

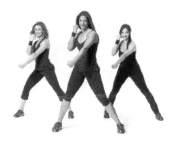

Bring your right fist back beside your chin and now powerfully punch your left fist down and diagonally across your body, allowing your torso to rotate to the left. Keep your elbows close to your sides and bring both fists back to either side of your chin after each punch.

Move with confidence. The important thing is not to achieve perfection but to be willing to improve. Every time you do one more than you want to, you have succeeded. Every time you get yourself out of your comfort zone, you have succeeded. The more you bend your knees, the more your legs will have to work. The more you twist during the punches, the more you will feel your abs working. Go for it!

Rhythm check: 4 counts

- "Until"—punch up to the right
- "I"—punch up to the left
- "Succeed"—punch down to the right
- [Beat/voice hold]—punch down to the left

Run through for 1 minute:

- "I will not stop"—4 counts
- "Until I succeed"—4 counts (up/up, down/down, alternating left and right)

Then run through from the top for another minute:

- "Yes!"—4 counts
- "This I must achieve"—4 counts
- "I will not stop"—4 counts
- "Until I succeed"—4 counts (up/up, down/down, alternating left and right)

INSPIRED

SAY, "I AM INSPIRED NOW."

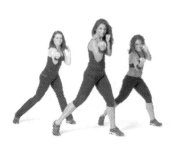

Stand with your feet hip width apart, your elbows bent and close to your body, your fists at either side of your chin, in the On-Guard position. Keeping your elbows bent, punch your right fistup toward the center of your body, allowing your torso to rotate slightly to the left. Return to the On-Guard position.

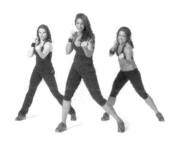

Repeat on the other side. Punch your left fist toward the center of your body, allowing your torso to rotate to the right. Remember to return to the On-Guard position after each punch.

Rhythm check: 8 counts
- "I"—uppercut punches to the right and left
- "am"—uppercut punches to the right and left
- "inspired"—uppercut punches to the right and left
- "now"—uppercut punches to the right and left

Do this for one minute, then go back to the top for one minute.

While you are doing this move, imagine how you would move if you were totally inspired. If you really wanted to give your all, how would you show it here? It is not the action but the spirit of the action that influences change. Be inspiring when you do this!

STRENGTH

SAY, "I AM STRONG ENOUGH."

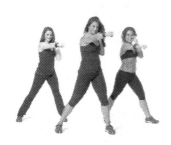

Stand with your feet hip width apart, your elbows bent and close to your body, your fists at either side of your chin, in the On-Guard position. Punch your right fist across your body, your palm facing down, allowing your torso to rotate slightly. Return to the On-Guard position.

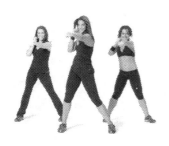

Repeat on the other side. Remember to keep your elbows pointing toward the floor and your palms facing down. Return to the On-Guard position after each punch.

Rhythm check: 8 counts
- "I"—punch right and left
- "am"—punch right and left
- "strong"—punch right and left
- "enough"—punch right and left

Run through for 1 minute:
- "I am inspired now"—8 counts
- "I am strong enough"—8 counts

CONFIDENCE

SAY, "I AM NEVER GIVING UP!"

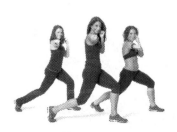

Stand in the On-Guard position. Pivot to your left, bending your knees in a lunge position (keep your left foot flat on the floor and allow your right heel to come off), and punch your right fist 2 times in a double punch toward center.

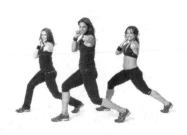

In one motion, pivot to the right and repeat on the other side, punching your left fist two times in a double punch toward center. Fully extend each arm in the double punch and return your arms to the On-Guard position after each double punch.

Rhythm check: 8 counts
- "I"—double punch to the right
- "am"—double punch to the left
- "never giving"—double punch right
- "up"—double punch left

Run through for one minute:
- "I am inspired now"—8 counts
- "I am strong enough"—8 counts
- "I am never giving up"—8 counts (two times right and left)

Put everything you have into this section! Feel the burning in your shoulders and arms. This series takes courage, and if you do it with your heart and soul and with the intention to build your warrior spirit, it will work! Challenge yourself! Don't do less than you can do! By the end of one minute, you should need a break!

Run through from the top (1–5 minutes):

- "Yes"—COMMITMENT (4 counts)
- "This I must achieve"—DESIRE (4 counts)
- "I will not stop"—VICTORY (4 counts)
- "Until I succeed"—FAITH (4 counts) (up/up, down/down, alternating left and right)
- "I am inspired now"—INSPIRED (8 counts)
- "I am strong enough"—STRENGTH (8 counts)
- "I am never giving up!"—CONFIDENCE (8 counts) (two times right and left)

WHEN YOU ARE TIRED / NEED ENERGY

I am strong now, I can handle this.
I am confident now, I can handle this.
I have willpower now, I can handle this.
I am accepting now, I can handle this.
Yes! Yes! Yes! Yes!
I want it, I want it, I really, really want it!
I believe I will succeed.

When you feel tired or need more energy, remember that disempowering thoughts deplete your energy and positive thoughts, whereas exercise increases your energy and releases endorphins—the "feel-good" chemicals in your body. Exercise and a positive attitude lead to more of the same. Get up and get going with this series. Don't wait to have the energy to do the series; do the series when you want to increase your energy. That is the warrior spirit!

STRENGTH

SAY, "I AM STRONG NOW"

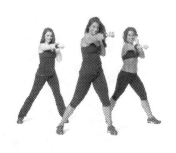

Stand with your feet hip width apart, your elbows bent and close to your body, your fists at either side of your chin, in the On-Guard position. Punch your right fist across your body, your palm facing down, allowing your torso to rotate slightly. Return to the On-Guard position.

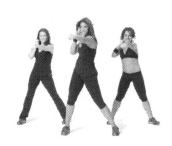

Repeat on the other side. Remember to keep your elbows pointing toward the floor and your palms facing down. Return to the On-Guard position after each punch.

SAY "I AM STRONG NOW, I CAN HANDLE THIS" FOR ONE MINUTE.

Rhythm check: 8 counts each affirmation
- "I"—punch right and left
- "am"—punch right and left
- "strong"—punch right and left
- "now"—punch right and left
- "I"—punch right and left
- "can"—punch right and left
- "handle"—punch right and left
- "this"—punch right and left

CONFIDENCE

SAY, "I AM CONFIDENT NOW"

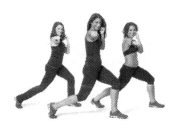

Stand in the On-Guard position. Pivot to your left, bending your knees in a lunge position (keep your left foot flat on the floor and allow your right heel to come up), and punch your right fist 2 times in a double punch toward center.

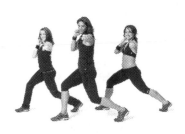

In one motion, pivot to the right and repeat on the other side, punching your left fist 2 times in a double punch toward center. Fully extend each arm in the double punch and return your arms to the On-Guard position after each double punch.

SAY "I AM CONFIDENT NOW, I CAN HANDLE THIS" FOR ONE MINUTE.

Rhythm check: 8 counts each affirmation
- "I"—double punch to the right
- "am"—double punch to the left
- "confident"—double punch right
- "now"—double punch left
- "I"—double punch to the right

- "can"—double punch to the left
- "handle"—double punch to the right
- "this"—double punch to the left

Run through for one minute:
- "I am strong now, I can handle this"—8 counts (4 sets of single punches right and left)
- "I am confident now, I can handle this"—8 counts (4 sets of double punches right and left)

KARMA (LEFT)

SAY, "I HAVE WILLPOWER NOW, I CAN HANDLE THIS."

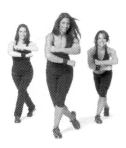

Step to the left and cross your right leg behind you, keeping your right heel off the ground. Your knees are bent, and your hips are square to the center. With your hands in fists and your elbows bent in front of you, roll your arms *away* from your body as fast as you can. Make sure your back is straight and your chest is open.

Rhythm check: 8 counts (for one minute)
- "I have willpower now, I can handle this"—hold the legs in the crossed position as the arms roll away from you for 8 counts.

You can handle anything. You are never given a challenge that you don't have the ability to handle.

KARMA (RIGHT)

SAY, "I AM ACCEPTING NOW, I CAN HANDLE THIS."

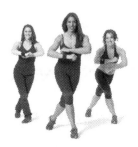 Now step to the right and cross your left leg behind you, keeping your right heel off the ground. Your knees are bent and your hips are square to the center. Keeping your arms where they are, roll them *toward* you as fast as you can. Make sure your back is straight and your chest is open.

Rhythm check: 8 counts (for one minute)
- "I am accepting now, I can handle this"—hold the legs in the crossed position as the arms roll away from you for 8 counts.

Run through for one minute: left and right for 8 counts each side
- "I have willpower now, I can handle this"
- "I am accepting now, I can handle this"

Run through from the top: run through for one minute:
- "I am strong now, I can handle this"—STRENGTH (8 counts, strong, single alternating punches)
- "I am confident now, I can handle this"—CONFIDENCE (8 counts, double alternating punches)
- "I have willpower now, I can handle this"—KARMA (LEFT) (8 counts, cross your right leg behind the left and your circle arms away from you)
- "I am accepting now, I can handle this"—KARMA (RIGHT) (8 counts, cross your left leg behind the right and your circle arms toward you)

The more you bend your knees in this exercise, the more you will work your legs. Do your best to hold it for one minute, and generate as much speed with the circling of your arms as you can.

COMMITMENT

SAY, "YES!" FOR ONE MINUTE, ALTERNATING LEFT AND RIGHT

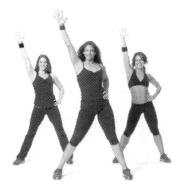

Stand with your feet more than shoulder width apart. Reach your right arm straight up over your head while slightly bending your right knee. Keep your left arm bent at your side. Both palms are facing forward.

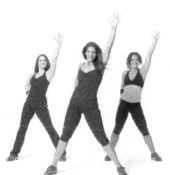

Now switch your arms, reaching your left arm straight up over your head while slightly bending your left knee. Now keep your right arm bent by your side. Both palms are facing forward.

Rhythm check: 8 counts

- Say "Yes!" every time the left arm extends to the sky.

Commit to the movement and embody the joy of saying yes!

DESIRE

SAY, "I WANT IT, I WANT IT, I REALLY, REALLY WANT IT!"

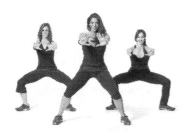

Assume the Warrior stance. Your hands are in front of you, with your thumbs and index fingers touching to create a triangle in front of your heart.

Remain in the Warrior stance. Keeping the triangle mudra with your hands, passionately extend your arms from your heart center.

Rhythm check:

- "I want it"—extend the arms out and back in 2 times
- "I want it"—extend the arms out and back in 2 times
- "I really, really"—extend the arms out and back in 2 times
- "want it!"—extend the arms out and back in 2 times

Run through for 1 minute:

- "Yes"—8 counts (say "yes" 4 times)
- "I want it, I want it, I really, really want it!"—8 counts

FAITH

SAY, "I BELIEVE I WILL SUCCEED."

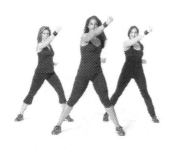

Stand with your feet hip width apart. Bend your elbows with your fists at either side of your chin. Powerfully punch your right fist up and diagonally across your body, allowing your torso to rotate to the left.

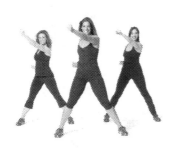

Bring your right fist back beside your chin and now powerfully punch your left fist up and diagonally across your body, allowing your torso to rotate to the right. Keep your elbows close to your sides and bring both fists back to either side of your chin after each punch.

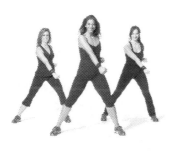

With your knees bent, powerfully punch your right fist down and diagonally across your body, allowing your torso again to rotate to the left. Make sure to keep your back straight and your abs in as you punch down.

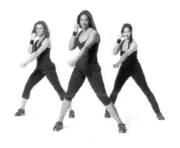

Bring your right fist back beside your chin and now powerfully punch your left fist down and diagonally across your body, allowing your torso to rotate to the left. Keep your elbows close to your sides and bring both fists back to either side of your chin after each punch.

This is a time to put your mind on your intention: See it, feel it, and be it. Declare out loud that you really want it, and let the fire of desire ignite your commitment to achieving it!

Rhythm check: 8 counts
- "I"—punch up to the right and left
- "believe"—punch down to the right and left
- "I will"—punch up to the right and left
- "succeed"—punch down to the right and left

Run through for one minute:
- "Yes"—8 counts (say "yes" 4 times)
- "I want it, I want it, I really, really want it!"—8 counts
- "I believe I will succeed"—8 counts

Final run-through from the top: 1–5 minutes

- "I am strong now, I can handle this"—STRENGTH (8 counts, single alternating punches)
- "I am confident now, I can handle this"—CONFIDENCE (8 counts, double alternating punches)
- "I have willpower now, I can handle this"—KARMA (8 counts, cross your right foot behind your left and circle arms toward you)
- "I am accepting now, I can handle this"—KARMA (8 counts, cross your left foot behind your right and circle arms away from you)
- "Yes"—COMMITMENT (8 counts—say "yes" 4 times, alternate arms reaching up)
- "I want it, I want it, I really, really want it!"—DESIRE (8 counts, passionately extend your arms from your heart)
- "I believe I will succeed"—FAITH (8 counts, punch up/ up, down/down)

This is a long series, and if you put your heart into it you will feel the energy building in you. Do this with the intention to build your power, your power to choose whom to be and how to live your life. You can do it!

IF YOU ARE FEELING TEMPTED

I have willpower now.
All negative thoughts stop right now.
I am unstoppable now.
Watch me.
I have faith now.
Temptation, so what! I'm ready to succeed.
Temptation, so what! I'm willing to succeed.
Temptation, so what! I'm able to succeed.
No matter what! I'm succeeding right now.
Yes! I am committed! Yes!
I like it, I like it, I really, really like it!

Temptation will always be around you, but when you are strong in your commitment, it will be easier to turn your eyes away from temptation and onto the goal. Every time you are tempted to give in or give up, know that every time you stick to your plan you will feel really good! It is empowering to keep your commitments because you gain trust in yourself. That is priceless! Hang in there, and when you give in to temptation, at least enjoy it fully. Drop the guilt and get back into the game! That's the warrior spirit! No regrets.

WILLPOWER

SAY, "I HAVE WILLPOWER NOW."

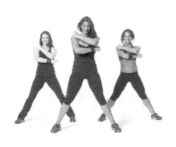

Your legs are straight in a wide V-stance; make sure to keep your back straight and your abs in. With your hands in fists and elbows bent in front of you, roll your arms *away* from your body as fast as you can (you can bend your knees if you want, to increase the intensity).

Rhythm check: 8 counts
- "I have willpower now"—stay in knee bend and roll arms for 8 counts (keep legs straight and roll arms for 8 counts)

SELF-CONTROL

SAY, "ALL NEGATIVE THOUGHTS STOP RIGHT NOW."

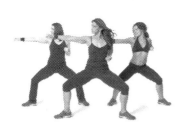

Stand in a straight-leg Warrior stance with your right forearm over your left forearm in front of your body, in the Chamber position. In one motion, bend your knees in the Warrior stance and open your arms, extending your right arm directly to your right side as the left fist slides back by your left shoulder, as if you are shooting a bow and arrow.

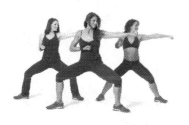

Return to the straight-leg Warrior stance and place your left forearm over your right forearm in front of your body in the Chamber position. Again, in one motion, bend your knees in the Warrior stance and open your arms, extending your left arm directly to your left side as the right fist slides back by your left shoulder, shooting a strong and powerful arrow.

Remember to keep the palm of your fist facing down to the floor as the arm extends, and don't let it overextend behind you.

Rhythm check: 4 counts

- "All negative"—chamber arms (place your right fore arm over your left, fists resting on elbows) and extend right arm
- "thoughts"—chamber arms and extend left arm
- "stop"—chamber arms and extend right arm
- "right now"—chamber arms and extend left arm

Run through for one minute:

- "I have willpower now"—4 counts
- "All negative thoughts stop right now"—4 counts

STRENGTH

SAY, "I AM UNSTOPPABLE NOW."

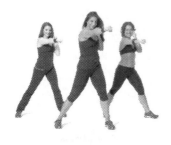

Stand with your feet hip width apart, your elbows bent and close to your body, your fists at either side of your chin, in the On-Guard position. Punch your right fist across your body, your palm facing down, allowing your torso to rotate slightly. Return to the On-Guard position.

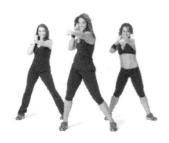

Repeat on the other side. Remember to keep your elbows pointing toward the floor and your palms facing down. Return to the On-Guard position after each punch.

Rhythm check: 8 counts for one minute
- "I"—punch right and left
- "am"—punch right and left
- "unstoppable"—punch right and left
- "now"—punch right and left

CONFIDENCE

SAY, "WATCH ME" (DOUBLE PUNCHES RIGHT AND LEFT FOR ONE MINUTE)

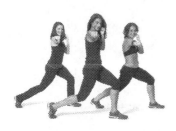

Stand in the On-Guard position. Pivot to your left, bending your knees in a lunge position (keep your left foot flat on the floor and allow your right heel to come up), and punch your right fist 2 times in a double punch toward center.

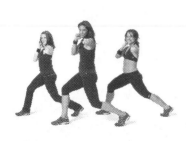

In one motion, pivot to the right and repeat on the other side, punching your left fist two times in a double punch toward center. Fully extend each arm in the double punch, and return your arms to the On-Guard position after each double punch.

Rhythm check: 8 counts
- "Watch me"—double punch to the right
- Voice hold (silence) —double punch to the left
- "Watch me"—double punch right
- Voice hold—double punch left

Run through for one minute:

- ▪ "I am unstoppable now"—8 counts (single alternating punches)
- ▪ "Watch me"—8 counts (4 sets of double punches right and left)

Then run through from the top for one minute:

- ▪ "I have willpower now"—WILLPOWER (8 counts, circle arms away from you)
- ▪ "All negative thoughts stop right now"—SELF-CON-TROL (8 counts, alternating blocks)
- ▪ "I am unstoppable now"—STRENGTH (8 counts, alternating single punches)
- ▪ "Watch me"—CONFIDENCE (8 counts, 4 sets of double punches right and left) (alternating double punches)

FAITH

SAY, "I HAVE FAITH NOW."

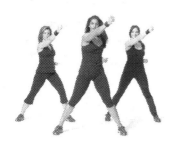

Stand with your feet hip width apart. Bend your elbows with your fists at either side of your chin. Powerfully punch your right fist up and diagonally across your body, allowing your torso to rotate to the left.

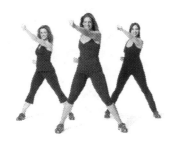

Bring your right fist back beside your waist and now powerfully punch your left fist up and diagonally across your body, allowing your torso to rotate to the right. Keep your elbows close to your sides and bring both fists back to either side of your chin after each punch.

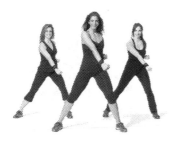

With your knees bent, powerfully punch your right fist down and diagonally across your body, allowing your torso to rotate to the left. Make sure to keep your back straight and your abs in as you punch down.

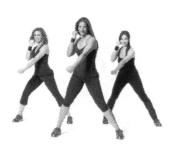

Bring your right fist back beside your chin and now powerfully punch your left fist down and diagonally across your body, allowing your torso to rotate to the left. Keep your elbows close to your sides and bring both fists back to either side of your chin after each punch.

Rhythm check: 8 counts
- "I"—punch up to the right and left
- "have"—punch down to the right and left
- "faith"—punch up to the right and left
- "now"—punch down to the right and left

From the top for one minute:
- "I have willpower now"—WILLPOWER (8 counts, circle arms away from you)
- "All negative thought stop right now"—SELF-CONTROL (8 counts, single alternating blocks)
- "I am unstoppable now"—STRENGTH (8 counts, alternating single punches)
- "Watch me"—CONFIDENCE (8 counts, alternating double punches)
- "I have faith now"—FAITH (8 counts, punch up/up, down/down)

READY TO TAKE ACTION

**SAY, "TEMPTATION, SO WHAT?
I'M READY TO SUCCEED."**

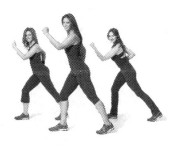

Pivot to the right and take a runner's stance, as if you were just about to take off in a sprint. Slightly bend your right knee, keeping your right foot flat on the floor and your left heel raised. Your elbows are bent, with your right arm in front of your body and the left arm behind you.

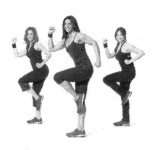

Like a spring, straighten your right leg and bring your left foot to meet your right knee. Switch your arm position as your knee comes up. Feel as if you are really taking off.

Rhythm check: 8 counts
- "Temptation, so what?"—raise left knee 2 times
- "I'm ready to succeed"—continue raising left knee 2 times

WILLING

SAY, "TEMPTATION, SO WHAT? I'M WILLING TO SUCCEED."

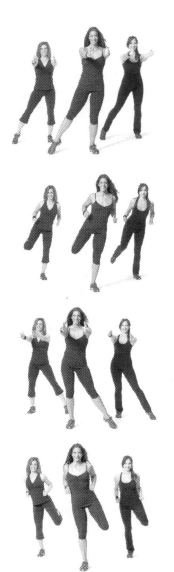

Step to the center with your left foot. Extend your arms parallel to the floor in front of you, shoulder width apart, with your palms facing.

Bend your right knee behind you and kick your butt with your heel. At the same time, slice your arms down by your sides with your elbows bent.

Now step your right foot down. Once again, extend your arms parallel to the floor and shoulder width apart with your palms facing.

Repeating the same move on the other side, bend your left knee behind you and kick your butt with your heel. At the same time, pull your arms down by your sides with bent elbows.

Rhythm check: 8 counts

- "Temptation, so what"—kick your butt right and left

- "I'm willing to succeed"—continue kicking your butt 2 times

ABLE

SAY, "TEMPTATION, SO WHAT?
I'M ABLE TO SUCCEED."

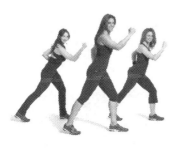

Pivot to your left and take a runner's stance. Now slightly bend your left knee, keeping your left foot flat on the floor and your right heel raised. Your elbows are bent, with your right arm in front of your body and your left arm behind you.

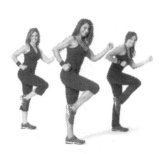

Like a spring, straighten your left leg and bring your right foot to meet your right knee. Switch your arm position as your knee comes up. Really feel as if you are taking off.

Rhythm check: 8 counts
- ■ "Temptation, so what"—raise right knee 2 times
- ■ "I'm able to succeed"—continue raising right knee 2 times

NOW

SAY, "NO MATTER WHAT, I'M SUCCEEDING RIGHT NOW."

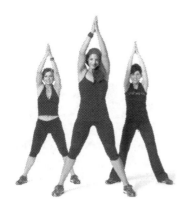

Do jumping jacks for one minute.

Rhythm check: 8 counts
- "No matter what"—2 jumping jacks (4 counts)
- "I'm succeeding right now"—2 jumping jacks (4 counts)

Run through for one minute:
- "Temptation, so what? I'm ready to succeed"—READY (8 counts)
- "Temptation, so what? I'm willing to succeed"—WILLING (8 counts)
- "Temptation, so what? I'm able to succeed"—ABLE (8 counts)
- "No matter what? I'm succeeding right now"—NOW (8 counts)

COMMITMENT

SAY, "YES! I AM COMMITTED! YES!"

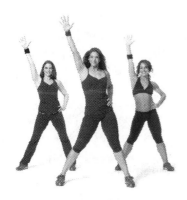

Stand with your feet more than shoulder width apart. Reach your right arm straight up over your head while slightly bending your right knee. Keep your left arm bent at your side. Both palms are facing forward.

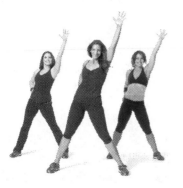

Now switch your arms, reaching your left arm straight up over your head while slightly bending your left knee. Keep your right arm bent by your side. Both palms are facing forward.

Rhythm check: 8 counts for one minute
- "Yes! I am committed! yes!"—alternate extended arms right and left

DESIRE

SAY, "I LIKE IT, I LIKE IT, I REALLY, REALLY LIKE IT!"

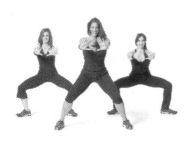

Assume the Warrior stance. Your hands are in front of you, with your thumbs and index fingers touching to create a triangle in front of your heart. Remain in the Warrior stance. Keeping the triangle mudra with your hands, passionately extend your arms from your heart center.

Rhythm check:

- "I like it"—extend the arms out and back in 2 times
- "I like it"—extend the arms out and back in 2 times
- "I really, really"—extend the arms out and back in 2 times
- "like it"—extend the arms out and back in 2 times

Run through for one minute:

- "Yes"—8 counts (say "yes" 4 times)
- "I like it, I like it, I really, really like it!"—8 counts

Run through from the top for one to five minutes:

- "I have willpower now"—WILLPOWER (8 counts, circle arms away from you)
- "All negative thoughts stop right now"—SELF-CONTROL (8 counts, single alternating blocks)
- "I am unstoppable now"—STRENGTH (8 counts, alternating single punches)
- "Watch me"—CONFIDENCE (8 counts, alternating double punches)
- "I have faith now"—FAITH (8 counts, punch up/up, down/down)
- "Temptation, so what? I'm ready to succeed"—READY (8 counts, bring your left knee up and down)
- "Temptation, so what? I'm willing to succeed"—WILLING (8 counts, alternating heel kicks to your buttock)
- "Temptation, so what? I'm able to succeed"—ABLE (8 counts, right knee up and down)
- "No matter what, I'm succeeding right now"—NOW (8 counts, jumping jacks)
- "Yes! I am committed! Yes!"—COMMITMENT (8 counts, alternating reaches)
- "I like it, I like it, I really, really like it!"—DESIRE (8 counts, passionately extend arms out and in)

It will take physical and mental endurance to get through the whole thing. Memorize it, embody it, and it will work. Just attack it as one move at a time, one affirmation at a time, one day at a time, and you will feel yourself becoming stronger and stronger. You will be able to face temptation. It just takes practice, desire, and belief!

WHEN YOU ARE STARVING

All I need is within me now.
I have the power to choose it
I have the power to use it
I am safe to feel
And accept I am now healed.

EMBRACE

SAY, "ALL"

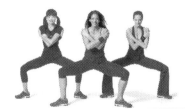

Step to the right into Warrior legs and give yourself a big hug.

POSITIVE EXPECTATION

SAY, "I NEED"

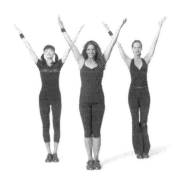

Step the right foot back to feet together. Extend your arms overhead in a V-position, your fingers wide, and look up to the sky.

EMBRACE

SAY, "IS WITHIN"

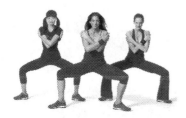

Step to the left into Warrior legs and give yourself a big hug.

POSITIVE EXPECTATION

SAY, "ME NOW."

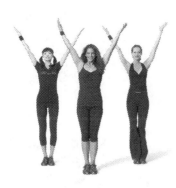

Step the left foot back to feet together. Extend your arms overhead in a V-position, your fingers wide, and look up to the sky.

Repeat and alternate right and left for one minute.

POWER

SAY, "I HAVE THE POWER"

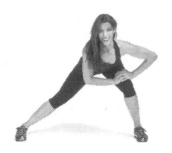

Take a wide step to the left in a deep, powerful lunge, bending your left knee deeply and keeping your right knee straight. Your back is straight your and your feet are parallel. Place both hands on your left thigh for support.

CHOOSE

SAY, "TO CHOOSE IT"

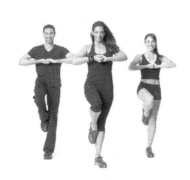

Push off your right foot to feet together. Now balance on your left leg with your right foot by your left knee. Bend your elbows and link your palms by bending your fingers in front of your heart, in the "choose" mudra. Pull your hands away from each other by activating your upper back muscles.

Repeat the same movements on the left side.

POWER

SAY, "I HAVE THE POWER"

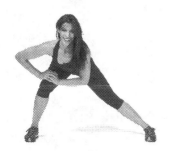

Take a wide step to the right in a deep powerful lunge, bending your right knee deeply and keeping your left knee straight. Your back is straight, and your feet are parallel. Place both hands on your right thigh for support.

CHOOSE

SAY, "TO USE IT"

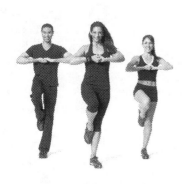

Push off your right foot to feet together. Now balance on your left leg with your right foot by your left knee. Bend your elbows and link your palms (remember to switch your hands!) by bending your fingers in front of your heart, in the "choose" mudra. Pull your hands away from each other by activating your upper back muscles.

Alternate right and left for one minute.

LOVE

SAY, "I AM SAFE"

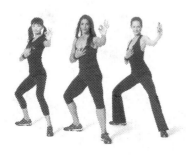

Step diagonally to the back with your right foot into the Warrior stance. Create two circles by touching your thumbs and index fingers. Place your right palm over your heart, extend your left arm forward, and gaze through the circle as through a keyhole.

COMPASSION

SAY, "TO FEEL"

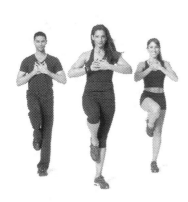

Stand on your left leg, your right foot by your left knee, in a single-leg balance. Place your palms over your heart.

Repeat the same movements on the left side.

LOVE

SAY, "AND ACCEPT"

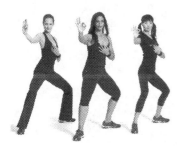

Step diagonally to the back with your left foot into the Warrior stance. Create two circles by touching your thumbs and index fingers. Place your left palm over your heart, extend your right arm forward, and gaze through the circle as through a keyhole.

COMPASSION

SAY, "I AM NOW HEALED."

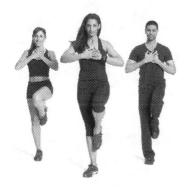

Stand on your right leg, your left foot by your right knee, in a single-leg balance. Place your palms over your heart.

Alternate right and left for one minute.

Put all three together just on the right side for one minute.

Put all three together on the left side for one minute.

Alternate right and left for three minutes.

WHEN YOU FEEL LIKE GIVING UP

One day at a time is really just fine.
I have the power to choose, and I never lose.
My life is a choice, I choose to rejoice.
With strength and compassion, I will take one action.

GRACE

SAY, "ONE DAY"

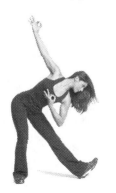

Stand with your feet together. Step and bend your right leg back and bow over your left leg, with your leg straight and your foot flexed. Sweep both arms back to your right side and bow deeply. Touch your thumbs and index fingers to create circles, and place your left hand over your heart.

READY

SAY, "AT A TIME"

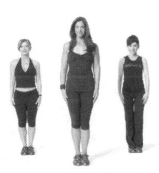

Step your right foot back to feet together, your arms by your sides, looking straight ahead in the Ready position.

Repeat the same movements on the left side.

GRACE

SAY, "IS REALLY"

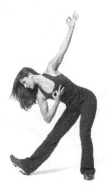

From the Ready position, step and bend your left leg back and bow over your right leg, with your leg straight and your foot flexed. Sweep both arms back to your left side and bow deeply. Touch your thumbs and index fingers to create a circle, and place your right hand over your heart.

READY

SAY, "JUST FINE."

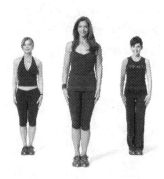

Step your left foot back to feet together, your arms by your sides, looking straight ahead in the Ready position.

POWER

SAY, "I HAVE THE POWER"

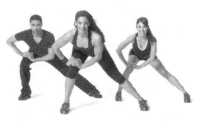

Take a wide step to the right in a deep, powerful lunge, bending your right knee deeply and keeping your left knee straight. Your back is straight, and your feet are parallel. Place both hands on your right thigh for support.

CHOOSE

SAY, "TO CHOOSE"

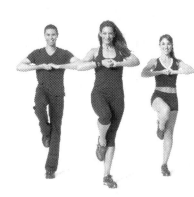

Push off your right foot to feet together. Now balance on your left leg with your right foot by your left knee. Bend your elbows and link your palms by bending your fingers in front of your heart. Pull your hands away from each other by activating your upper back muscles.

Repeat the same movements on the left side.

POWER

SAY, "AND I"

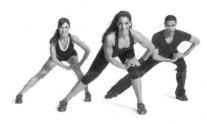

Take a wide step to the left in a deep, powerful lunge, bending your left knee deeply and keeping your right knee straight. Your back is straight, and yourfeet are parallel. Place both hands on your left thigh for support.

CHOOSE

SAY, "NEVER LOSE."

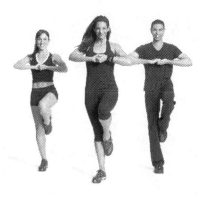

Push off your left foot to feet together. Now balance on your right leg with your left foot by your right knee. Bend your elbows and link your palms (remember to switch your hands!) by bending your fingers in front of your heart. Pull your hands away from each other by activating your upper back muscles.

Alternate right and left for one minute.

SAY, "MY LIFE IS A CHOICE"

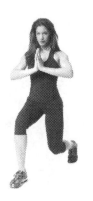

Stand with your feet together and your palms pressed together over your heart, in the Prayer position. Take a large step forward with your right foot and bend your knees to a front lunge, keeping your front foot flat on the floor and your knee tracking over your ankle. Allow the heel of your left foot to come off the floor. Tuck your pelvis under while keeping your back straight and your abs in.

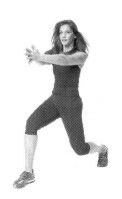

Remain in the front lunge position and extend your arms straight out in front of you, palms pressed together.

ACCEPTANCE

SAY, "I CHOOSE TO REJOICE"

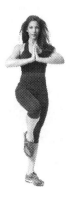

Pushing off from your right foot, step back to feet together or into a single-leg balance, bringing your right foot to your left knee. Return your arms to the Prayer position, your palms together over your heart.

Repeat the same movements on the left side.

FEARLESS

SAY, "WITH STRENGTH AND COMPASSION"

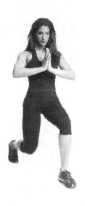

Stand with your feet together and your palms pressed together over your heart, in the Prayer position. Take a large step forward with your left foot and bend your knees to a front lunge, keeping your front foot flat on the floor and your knee tracking over your ankle. Allow the heel of your right foot to come off the floor. Tuck your pelvis under while keeping your back straight and yourabs in.

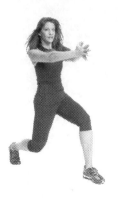

Remain in the front lunge position and extend your arms straight out in front of you, palms pressed together.

ACCEPTANCE

SAY, "I WILL TAKE ONE ACTION."

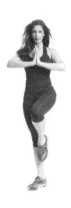

Pushing off from your left foot, step back to feet together or into a single-leg balance, bringing your left foot to your right knee. Return your arms to the Prayer position, your palms together over your heart.

Alternate right and left for one minute.

WHEN THE SCALE REFUSES TO BUDGE

I'm a warrior, and I'm ready.
I have willpower.
I have strength.
I have faith.
It's on its way
I am positive now!
I am ready to feel good
I am willing to feel good
I am able to feel good
I am feeling better now!

If the scale is refusing to budge, maybe you need to take your attention off the scale for a while and observe if you are sabotaging your efforts by not believing in yourself. Remind yourself that if you stick with it, and if you do something (anything!) differently than you have before, things will change. Are you really willing to feel good? Don't let your happiness depend on the number on the scale. Stick to your plan, honestly do your best, and be willing to feel better now.

WARRIOR

SAY, "I'M A WARRIOR"

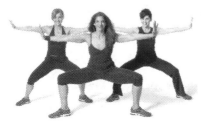

From a standing position, jump to a wide bent-knee V-stance, keeping your knees over your ankles. Simultaneously extend your arms to either side of your body and flex your wrists. Keep your back straight, your abs in.

READINESS

SAY, "AND I'M READY"

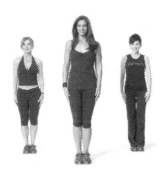

Jump your feet together, standing tall, and bring your arms by your sides.

Rhythm check: 8 counts

- "I'm a warrior"—4 counts
- "And I'm ready"—4 counts

PATRICIA MORENO

WILLPOWER

SAY, "I HAVE WILLPOWER."

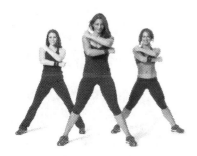

Jump or step your feet to a wide V-stance and bend your knees. With your hands in fists and your elbows bent in front of you, roll your arms *away* from your body as fast as you can, going into a deep knee bend.

Rhythm check: 4 counts

- "I have willpower"—stay in knee bend and roll arms for 4 counts

STRENGTH

SAY, "I HAVE STRENGTH."

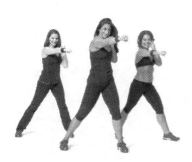

Stand with your feet hip width apart, your elbows bent and close to your body, your fists at either side of your chin, in the On-Guard position. Punch your right fist across your body, your palm facing down, allowing your torso to rotate slightly. Return to the On-Guard position.

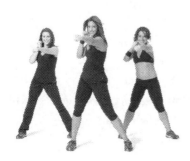

Repeat on the other side. Remember to keep your elbows pointing toward the floor and your palms facing down. Return to the On-Guard position after each punch.

Rhythm check: 4 counts
- "I have"—punch right and left
- "strength"—punch right and left

Run through for one minute:
- "I have willpower"—stay in knee bend and roll arms for 4 counts
- "I have strength"—4 counts

FAITH

SAY, "I HAVE FAITH."

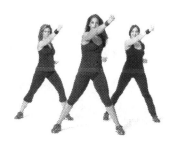

Stand with your feet hip width apart. Bend your elbows with your fists at either side of your chin. Powerfully punch your right fist up and diagonally across your body, allowing your torso to rotate to the left.

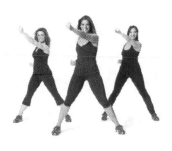

Bring your right fist back beside your chin and now powerfully punch your left fist up and diagonally across your body, allowing your torso to rotate to the right. Keep your elbows close to your sides and bring both fists back to either side of your chin after each punch.

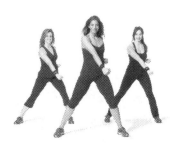

With your knees bent, powerfully punch your right fist down and diagonally across your body, allowing your torso to rotate to the left. Make sure to keep your back straight and your abs in as you punch down.

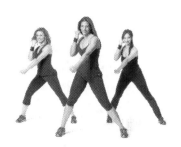

Bring your right fist back beside your chin and now powerfully punch your left fist down and diagonally across your body, allowing your torso to rotate to the right.

PATRICIA MORENO

GREAT

SAY, "IT'S ON ITS WAY"

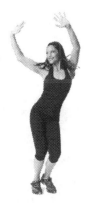

Pump your arms up and down overhead while jogging in place for one minute.

Rhythm check: 4 counts

- "It's on its"—arms up and down for 2 counts

- "way"—arms up and down for 2 counts

Run through for one minute:
- "I have faith now"—4 counts
- "It's on its way"—4 counts

Run through for another minute:
- "I have willpower"—WILLPOWER (stay in knee bend and roll arms for 4 counts)
- "I have strength"—STRENGTH (4 counts, single alternating punches)
- "I have faith now"—FAITH (4 counts, punch up/up, down/down)
- "It's on its way"—GREAT (4 counts)

This should feel like a celebration! You're raising the roof! You feel the excitement of knowing your success is on its way!

HAPPY

SAY, "I AM POSITIVE NOW!"

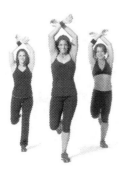

Circle your arms away from you in giant sweeping arcs as you alternate kicking each heel to your butt.

Rhythm check: 8 counts (4 arm circles)

- "I"—kick your butt with your left foot and circle your arms
- "am"—kick your butt with your right foot and circle your arms
- "positive"—kick your butt with your left foot and circle your arms
- "now"—kick your butt with your right foot and circle your arms

Run through from the top for one minute:

- "I'm a warrior and I'm ready"—WARRIOR READY (8 counts)
- "I have willpower"—WILLPOWER (stay in knee bend and roll arms for 4 counts)
- "I have strength"—STRENGTH (4 counts, single alternating punches)
- "I have faith"—FAITH (4 counts, punch up/up, down/down)
- "It's on its way"—GREAT (4 counts)
- "I am positive now"— HAPPY (8 counts) (4 arm circles)

This move generates a lot of energy in your body! The sweeping motion of the arms symbolizes your intention to gather all your positive power now! Enjoy it, be playful, be silly, be joyful. Add a big huge grin on your face on purpose and for no reason at all.

READY TO TAKE ACTION

SAY, "I AM READY TO FEEL GOOD"

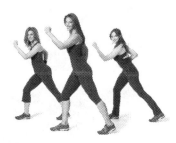

Pivot to the right and take a runner's stance, as if you were just about to take off in a sprint. Slightly bend your right knee, keeping your right foot flat on the floor and your left heel raised. Your elbows are bent, with your left arm in front of your body and your right arm behind you.

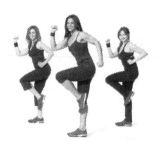

Like a spring, straighten your right leg and bring your left foot to meet the right knee. Switch your arm position as the knee comes up. Feel as if you are really taking off.

Rhythm check: 4 counts (2 knee raises/2 arm pumps)
- "I am ready"—raise left knee and switch arms back to front
- "to feel good"—raise left knee again and switch arms back to front

This is a great section to get your heart rate up!

WILLING

SAY, "I AM WILLING TO FEEL GOOD"

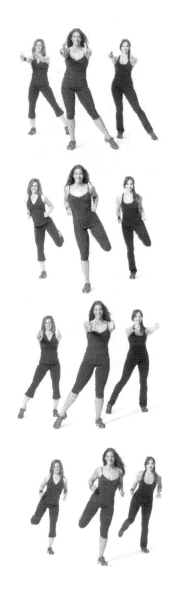

Step to the center with your left foot. Extend your arms parallel to the floor in front of you, shoulder width apart, with your palms facing.

Bend your right knee behind you and kick your butt with your heel. At the same time, slice your arms down by your sides with your elbows bent.

Now step your right foot down. Once again, extend your arms parallel to the floor and shoulder width apart with your palms facing.

Repeating the same move on the other side, bend your left knee behind you and kick your butt with your heel. At the same time, slice your arms down by your sides with bent elbows.

Rhythm check: 4 counts

- "I am willing"—(4 counts, kick your butt with your right foot, arms go up and down)

- "to feel good"—(4 counts, kick your butt with your right foot, arms go up and down)

ABLE

SAY, "I AM ABLE TO FEEL GOOD"

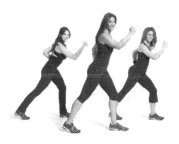

Now pivot to the left and take a runner's stance on the left side. Slightly bend your left knee, keeping your left foot flat on the floor and your right heel raised. Your elbows are bent, with your left arm in front of your body and your right arm behind you.

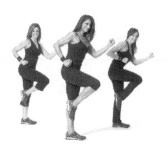

Like a spring, straighten your left leg and bring your right foot to meet the left knee. Switch your arm position as your knee comes up.

Rhythm check: 4 counts (2 knee raises/2 arm pumps)
- "I am able"—raise left knee and switch arms back to front
- "to feel good"—raise left knee again and switch arms back to front

NOW

SAY, "I AM FEELING BETTER NOW!" FOR ONE MINUTE.

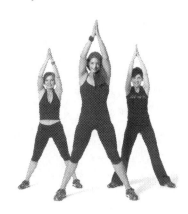

Do jumping jacks for one minute.

Rhythm check: 4 counts (2 jumping jacks)

- "I am feeling better"—1 jumping jack (2 counts)
- "right now"—1 jumping jack (2 counts)

Run through for one minute:

- I am ready to feel good—4 counts
- I am willing to feel good—4 counts
- I am able to feel good—4 counts
- I am feeling better now!—4 counts

Run through from the top for one minute:

- "I'm a warrior, and I'm ready"—WARRIOR-READINESS 8 counts
- "I have willpower"—WILLPOWER (4 counts, stay in knee bend and roll arms for 4 counts)
- "I have strength"—STRENGTH (4 counts, alternating straight punches)

- "I have faith"—FAITH (4 counts, alternating punches up/ up, down/down)
- "It's on its way!"—GREAT (raise the roof) (4 counts)
- "I am positive now"— HAPPY (8 counts) (4 arm circles) (4 arm circles)
- "I am ready to feel good"—READY TO TAKE ACTION (4 counts, raise left knee up and down and switch arms back to front)
- "I am willing to feel good"—WILLING (4 counts, alternating heel kicks to your buttocks)
- "I am able to feel good"—ABLE (4 counts, raise right knee up and down and switch arms back to front)
- "I am feeling better now!"—NOW (4 counts, jumping jacks)

Remember, progress feels good. It is never about perfection.

CHAPTER CHECKLIST
i Will . . .

✳ Look through the different workouts in this chapter and find one that inspires me.

✳ Do that series until I know it by heart and I don't have to look at the book.

✳ Do something every day that will help me improve my mood and my attitude.

ACKNOWLEDGMENTS

My heartfelt thanks to the many teachers, family, and friends who have all been a part of bringing this work together.

Thanks to:

My parents, who urged me to be who I wanted to be and to do what I wanted to do.

My sister, Norma, who embodies courage and faith when dealing with difficulty

My wife, Kellen, who helped me learn to love with all my heart. I love you

My teacher, John Friend of Anusara yoga, who deeply inspired me to create this method

My students, who have been daring enough to try new things

Lisa Jubilee, for her supportive and generous nutritional advice

Natalia Petrzela, who helped me clarify my thoughts and ideas

Kat Ademenko, for beautifully explaining each exercise in this book

Sheryl Berk, for all her hard work in making these pages beautifully come together with her talent for bringing the best out in me and then making it even better

Frank Weinman, my literary agent, who made it all come together

Lauren Zander and Laurie Gerber of the Handel Method, who constantly coached me to live out loud

Fernando Milani, for the beautiful pictures in this book

Helio de Souza for being the hairstylist for this shoot

Equinox fitness club for being the first gym in the United States to endorse this program.

ABOUT THE AUTHOR

Patricia Moreno has dedicated her life to empowering people all over the world to transform their bodies and their minds. Her creative blend of inspiration and power has kept her at the top of the international fitness scene for fifteen years. She has been featured in numerous magazines such as *Shape, Fitness*, and *Women's Health*. *New York* magazine named her Best Instructor in New York City, and *Shape* magazine named her one of the top ten women who shape the world. She was the fitness adviser for *Fitness* magazine and has trained thousands of instructors worldwide in her workout programs She has starred in and choreographed more than fifteen workout videos. Her fitness programs cross the line between personal empowerment and fitness as she blends her extensive training in dance, yoga, martial arts, and personal transformation technology. She lives and works in New York City and is invited to lead her workshops internationally.

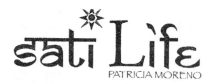

PATRICIA MORENO

Join the Sati Life community online
at www.satilife.com or at www.patriciamoreno.com.

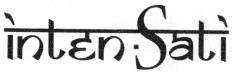

INTENTION · AWARENESS

Visit iTunes to download the IntenSati application to your
iPhone or your iPod Touch.

Please check out
www.iquest.com for
more of Patricia's workouts.

Printed in the United States
By Bookmasters